Workbook *for*

Understanding Pharmacology *for* Pharmacy Technicians

Mary Ann Stuhan, PharmD, RPh

Pharmacy Program Manager
Cuyahoga Community College
Cleveland, Ohio

American Society of Health-System Pharmacists®
Bethesda, Maryland

Any correspondence regarding this publication should be sent to the publisher, American Society of Health-System Pharmacists, 7272 Wisconsin Avenue, Bethesda, MD 20814, attention: Special Publishing.

The information presented herein reflects the opinions of the contributors and advisors. It should not be interpreted as an official policy of ASHP or as an endorsement of any product.

Because of ongoing research and improvements in technology, the information and its applications contained in this text are constantly evolving and are subject to the professional judgment and interpretation of the practitioner due to the uniqueness of a clinical situation. The editor and ASHP have made reasonable efforts to ensure the accuracy and appropriateness of the information presented in this document. However, any user of this information is advised that the editor and ASHP are not responsible for the continued currency of the information, for any errors or omissions, and/or for any consequences arising from the use of the information in the document in any and all practice settings. Any reader of this document is cautioned that ASHP makes no representation, guarantee, or warranty, express or implied, as to the accuracy and appropriateness of the information contained in this document and specifically disclaims any liability to any party for the accuracy and/or completeness of the material or for any damages arising out of the use or non-use of any of the information contained in this document.

Director, Special Publishing: Jack Bruggeman
Acquisitions Editor: Jack Bruggeman
Editorial Project Manager: Ruth Bloom
Production Editor: Johnna Hershey
Cover Design: David Wade
Page Design: David Wade

ISBN: 978-1-58528-383-5

CONTENTS

Preface.. v

Part 1: Introduction

Chapter 1 1
Why Technicians Need to Study Pharmacology and Therapeutics

Chapter 2 5
Pharmacokinetics

Part 2: The Nervous System

Chapter 3 7
The Autonomic Nervous System

Chapter 4 11
The Central Nervous System

Chapter 5 15
Neurologic Disorders

Chapter 6 19
Psychiatric Diseases

Part 3: The Endocrine System

Chapter 7 23
Overview of the Endocrine System and Agents

Chapter 8 27
Adrenal Gland Hormones

Chapter 9 31
Diabetes

Chapter 10 35
Reproductive Hormones

Part 4: The Musculoskeletal System and Related Topics

Chapter 11 39
Overview of the Musculoskeletal System

Chapter 12 43
Musculoskeletal Disorders

Part 5: The Cardiovascular and Renal Systems

Chapter 13 47
Overview of the Cardiovascular and Renal Systems

Chapter 14 51
Hypertension

Chapter 15 55
Heart Disease

Chapter 16 59
Hyperlipidemia

Part 6: The Respiratory System

Chapter 17 63
Overview of the Respiratory System

Chapter 18 65
Disorders of the Respiratory System

Part 7: The Gastrointestinal System

Chapter 19 69
Acid-Related Diseases of the Upper Gastrointestinal Tract

Chapter 20 73
Nausea, Vomiting, and Upper GI Tract Motility Disorders

Chapter 21 77
Lower Gastrointestinal Tract

Chapter 22 81
Hepatic and Pancreatic Disorders

Chapter 23 85
Nutritional Pharmacology

Part 8: The Hematologic System

Chapter 24 89
Overview of the Hematologic System

Chapter 25 91
Disorders of the Hematologic System

Part 9: Infectious Diseases

Chapter 26 95
Bacterial Infections

Chapter 27 101
Viral Infections

Chapter 28 105
Fungal Infections

Chapter 29 109
Immunobiologics

Part 10: Antineoplastic Agents

Chapter 30 113
Cancer

Part 11: The Dermatologic System

Chapter 31 117
Overview of the Skin and Topical Dosage Forms

Chapter 32 121
Treatment of Dermatologic Disorders

Part 12: Preparations for the Eye, Ear, Nose, and Throat

Chapter 33 127
Ophthalmic Medications

Chapter 34 131
Ear Medications

Chapter 35 133
Mouth, Throat, and Nose Medications

Answer Key.. 137

Preface

Pharmacology, an important area of study for everyone who handles medications in a healthcare setting, is especially critical for members of the pharmacy staff. Although *Understanding Pharmacology for Pharmacy Technicians* compiles vital pharmacology information, learning the drugs, their actions, and the terminology associated with the disease states being treated can seem like an overwhelming task. The *Workbook for Understanding Pharmacology for Pharmacy Technicians* has been designed to guide and assist students and pharmacy technicians toward a mastery of the knowledge and skills presented in the text.

Chapters in the *Workbook* are aligned with those in the text so that students and instructors can use it as a companion. Key concepts and pronunciations, along with the names, indications, and routes of administration of the medications covered in each chapter are emphasized in a variety of exercises including matching, true or false, and short answer questions. The range of exercises allows for use of the workbook to reinforce material presented in briefer, "overview" courses included in short-term curricula as well as its application to the more detailed learning required in lengthier, degree-granting programs. Students can use the workbook as a study guide for each chapter, and instructors can employ it as a resource for assignments and class exercises. Most workbook chapters include a drug monograph form, along with suggestions for the kinds of medications for which it might be useful in pharmacy practice situations. This drug monograph exercise affords students the chance and the method to study a medication in more detail, and learn how it compares to other therapies while giving them the opportunity to truly understand the pharmacology for a particular treatment area. It provides a way for instructors to demonstrate the application of pharmacology knowledge to development of a tool for making purchasing and formulary decisions.

Keeping in mind that ASHP's **Pharmacy Practice Model Initiative** (**PPMI**) includes advanced roles for pharmacy technicians with appropriate education, many students and instructors will wish to cover the material in greater depth. Toward this end, they can make use of the "additional study" suggestions, as well as rising to the challenge of using resources beyond the textbook to complete all parts of the drug monograph exercise.

At every level of educational plan, the *Understanding Pharmacology for Pharmacy Technicians* textbook and workbook package has been aimed at the meeting the goals of the **ASHP Accreditation Standard** and related knowledge areas (including medication safety, inventory management, and pharmacy law) of the **Pharmacy Technician Certification Board** (**PTCB**) examination. I hope that it will become a valuable resource in the education of twenty-first century pharmacy technicians.

Mary Ann Stuhan

March 2013

CHAPTER 1

Why Technicians Need to Study Pharmacology and Therapeutics

LEARNING OBJECTIVES

After completing this chapter, you should be able to

1. Define the terms drug, medication, pharmacology, and therapeutics and explain how they are related to one another and to pharmacy practice

2. Give reasons why it is essential for pharmacy technician students to learn pharmacology

3. Understand how pharmacology applies to the pharmacy technician's duties

4. Relate how the study of pharmacology contributes to professional development

5. Illustrate ways in which the technician's knowledge of pharmacology may be used to provide value to the pharmacist

6. Understand how pharmacology relates to patient safety

PRONUNCIATIONS

Homeostasis (hoe-mee-oh-STAY-sis)

Pharmaceutical (far-muh-SOO-tih-kul)

Pharmacology (far-muh-KOL-oh-jee)

Therapeutics (thayr-uh-PYOO-tikz)

Matching

Match each term to its definition.

DEFINITIONS

_____ 1. Agent used in the diagnosis, treatment, or prevention of disease

_____ 2. State of equilibrium of the internal environment of the body that is maintained by dynamic processes of feedback and regulation

_____ 3. Study of drugs

_____ 4. Study of expected results, dosages, side effects, and toxicities of agents used in the diagnosis, treatment, or prevention of disease

_____ 5. Study of the harmful effects of substances on the human body

_____ 6. Substance that may be expected to change or influence processes occurring in a living organism

TERMS

a. Drug
b. Homeostasis
c. Medication
d. Pharmacology
e. Therapeutics
f. Toxicology

True or False

For additional study, try to change the false statements to make them true.

_____1. The study of pharmacology is not related to other subjects.

_____2. Pharmaceutical is another term for a medication.

_____3. Pharmacy technicians must learn pharmacology but seldom use their knowledge of this subject at work.

_____4. It is important for pharmacy technicians to know which drugs are stored in particular areas of the pharmacy and why.

_____5. A knowledgeable pharmacy technician can have a more positive relationship with other healthcare providers.

_____6. Knowledge of pharmacology is unrelated to patient safety issues.

_____7. Pharmacy technicians deal only with pharmacists and customers.

_____8. Pharmacists have so many years of education that a pharmacy technician's knowledge is little additional help to them.

_____9. Knowing how drugs work can help a pharmacy technician better understand comments and questions from patients.

_____10. Knowledgeable pharmacy technicians can sometimes assume more interesting roles in patient care.

Short Answer

1. Read the case study at the beginning of Chapter 1 and describe how knowledge of pharmacology can help the technician do his or her job most effectively.

2. **Drug Monograph:** A drug monograph summarizes important information about a medication or a particular dosage form. Pharmacists, physicians, and insurance companies rely on the content of drug monographs in making decisions about which drugs to stock, prescribe, or recommend. Review the drug monograph that follows to find the answers to the questions below.

a. What do the terms *indication, contraindication,* and *adverse reaction* mean in the context of pharmacy?

b. What is a drug/food interaction?

c. What is meant by *Pregnancy Category,* and why is it important?

DRUG MONOGRAPH

Sample Drug Monograph

Generic Name   Atorvastatin

Brand Name   Lipitor

Manufacturer   Parke Davis

APPROVED INDICATION(S)

Hypercholesterolemia; prevention and risk reduction for coronary heart disease.

DOSAGE AND ROUTE(S) OF ADMINISTRATION

oral

AVAILABLE DOSAGE FORM(S) STRENGTH(S)

Tablet	10mg, 20mg, 40mg, 80mg

STORAGE/HANDLING CONDITIONS/PROCEDURES

Store at controlled room temperature (20° to 25°C [68° to 77°F])

PRECAUTIONS (CONTRAINDICATIONS, DRUG/FOOD INTERACTIONS, PREGNANCY CATEGORY)

Contraindications: Avoid use in active liver disease, elevated liver enzymes, hypersensitivity, pregnancy, breastfeeding.

Interactions: (Food) high-fiber foods may decrease absorption; grapefruit juice in large quantities may increase risk of side effects; alcohol in large quantities should be avoided.

Drugs: amiodarone, antacids, antifungals, some antibiotics, calcium channel blockers

Pregnancy Category X: Safety in pregnant women has not been established.

COMMON OR SEVERE ADVERSE REACTIONS

Common adverse reactions are gastro-intestinal (abdominal pain, constipation, dyspepsia, flatulence). Severe adverse reactions include liver toxicity and rhabdomyolysis (muscle breakdown).

INSTRUCTIONS FOR PATIENTS

Follow diet and exercise recommenda-tions; report any unexplained muscle pain to a healthcare practitioner; avoid pregnancy.

COST OF THERAPY (DAILY, MONTHLY, FULL COURSE)

$4.72 – $7.07 daily (wholesale price). Generics are available at wholesale prices of $0.52 - $5.49 daily

OTHER DRUGS IN THIS CLASS

fluvastatin, lovastatin, pravastatin, rosuvastatin, simvastatin

ADDITIONAL MEDICATIONS WITH SAME INDICATION

For hyperlipidemia: cholestyramine, colesevelam, colestipol, ezetimibe, niacin

ADVANTAGES/DISADVANTAGES COMPARED TO DRUGS LISTED ABOVE (CLASS, INDICATION)

Of the antihyperlipidemic agents, only atorvas-tatin is approved for use in prevention of cardio-vascular disease. Once daily administration is convenient. Availability of generics may reduce the price.

Compared to other categories of antihyperlipid-emics, drugs in this class pose a higher risk of liver disease and muscle injury.

CHAPTER 2

Pharmacokinetics

LEARNING OBJECTIVES

After completing this chapter, you should be able to

1. Define pharmacokinetics and relate its principles to the work of a pharmacy technician
2. Relate the route of administration to the actions of a drug and define at least eight routes of administration
3. Define absorption, distribution, metabolism, and excretion and the relevance of each to pharmacokinetic principles
4. Discuss how pharmacokinetics contributes to dosage regimens
5. Relate pharmacokinetic principles to the problem of drug interactions

PRONUNCIATIONS

Bioavailability (bie-oh-ah-VAY-luh-BIL-it-ee)

Genomic (gee-NO-mik)

Metabolism (meh-TAB-oh-lism)

Pharmacokinetics (far-muh-koe-ki-NET-ix)

Prodrug (PROH-drug)

Regimen (REJ-ih-men)

Matching I

Match each term to its definition.

DEFINITIONS

_____ 1. Change or breakdown of a drug by the body's enzymes

_____ 2. Drugs that have a large fraction of the active drug metabolized before reaching the systemic circulation

_____ 3. Elimination of the drug and/or its metabolites from the body

_____ 4. Fraction of the administered dose that is available to the systemic circulation

_____ 5. How much drug will be given how often

_____ 6. Method of giving a drug

_____ 7. Movement of a drug from systemic circulation to its points of concentration throughout the body

_____ 8. Movement of a drug from the point of administration into the systemic circulation

_____ 9. Point in therapy when the amount of drug administered exactly replaces the amount of drug removed

_____10. Range of drug concentrations for which the majority of patients show effective therapeutic response with minimal drug-related side effects

_____11. Study of the body's effect on a drug

_____12. Substance that must be converted into an active form by the body, usually by an enzyme

_____13. Time it takes for one half of the drug to be removed from the body

_____14. Volume of serum, plasma, or blood that has all of the drug removed per unit of time by the eliminating organ

TERMS

a. Absorption
b. Bioavailability
c. Clearance
d. Distribution
e. Dosage regimen
f. Excretion
g. First pass drugs
h. Half-life
i. Metabolism
j. Pharmacokinetics
k. Prodrug
l. Route of administration
m. Steady state
n. Therapeutic range

Matching II

Match each route of administration to its common abbreviation.

ROUTE OF ADMINISTRATION

_____1. Inhalation   _____5. Rectal

_____2. Intramuscular   _____6. Sublingual

_____3. Intravenous   _____7. Vaginal

_____4. Oral (by mouth)

ABBREVIATIONS

a.   IM   e.   PR

b.   INH   f.   PV

c.   IV   g.   SL

d.   PO

True or False

For additional study, try to change the false statements to make them true.

_____1.   Application of pharmacokinetics allows pharmacists and physicians to know exactly what effects a drug will have on a patient.

_____2.   Application of pharmacokinetics allows prediction and avoidance of some drug interactions.

_____3.   Medications are always administered by the route the patient prefers.

_____4.   Drugs administered by mouth must be absorbed from the gastrointestinal tract into the circulation to produce a systemic (body-wide) effect.

_____5.   Medications administered under the tongue take longer to produce an action than those that are swallowed.

_____6.   Topical application is the term used for medications administered by injection.

_____7.   Topical routes of administration deliver drugs in a way that does not require absorption from the gastrointestinal tract.

_____8.   Transdermal administration works only for drugs used to treat skin conditions.

_____9.   Dose regimen design takes into account pharmacokinetic principles to determine how much of and how often a drug should be administered.

_____10.   Drug interactions may involve the absorption, metabolism, or excretion of one or both of the drugs involved.

Short Answer

1. What benefit can the pharmacist achieve by applying pharmacokinetic principles to monitoring a patient's drug regimen? How are drug concentrations for this monitoring process determined?

2. What are metabolites, and how are they formed? What effects might they have on a patient?

Drug Monograph

Review the drug monograph at the end of Chapter 1 of this workbook and find the answers to the following questions.

1. By what route of administration do patients take atorvastatin? What does this mean?

2. How does the atorvastatin get from the route of entry into the body to the place where it acts?

3. What is the cause for concern about patients consuming high fiber foods?

CHAPTER 3

The Autonomic Nervous System

LEARNING OBJECTIVES

After completing this chapter, you should be able to

1. Define the autonomic nervous system (ANS) and its divisions, the parasympathetic and sympathetic autonomic nervous systems (PANS and SANS, respectively)

2. Outline the anatomy, physiology, and functions of the ANS, PANS, and SANS

3. Describe the targets/sites of action of endogenous neurotransmitters and of exogenous drugs that act on the ANS

4. Review the classification and mechanisms of action of drugs acting on the ANS

5. List therapeutic applications of the primary drug classes acting on the ANS

6. State the brand and generic names of representative therapeutic agents acting on the ANS, together with their routes of administration, side effects, and potential drug interactions

PRONUNCIATIONS

Adrenal (uh-DREE-nul)

Adrenergic (ADD-ren-ER-jik)

Autonomic (ot-oh-NOM-ik)

Catecholamine (kat-eh-KOL-uh-meen)

Cholinergic (kol-in-ER-jik)

Endocrine (EN-doh-krin)

Endogenous (en-DOJ-en-us)

Neuron (NYOOR-on)

Neurotransmitter (nyoor-oh-TRANZ-mit-er)

Parasympathetic (PAYR-uh-SIM-puh-THET-ik)

Sympathetic (SIM-puh-THET-ik)

Matching I

Match each body response to the sympathetic or parasympathetic nervous system by writing **SANS** *or* **PANS** *on the line to its left.*

_____ Bladder sphincter contraction

_____ Bladder sphincter relaxation

_____ Blood vessel constriction

_____ Blood vessel dilation

_____ Bronchoconstriction

_____ Bronchodilation

_____ Constriction of pupils (miosis)

_____ Decreased gland secretion

_____ Decreased gastrointestinal motility

_____ Decreased heart rate

_____ Dilation of pupils (mydriasis)

_____ Increased gastrointestinal motility

_____ Increased gland secretion

_____ Increased heart rate

Matching II

Match each brand name antimuscarinic medication to its generic name. For additional study, use the space next to the medication to write the indications for each drug.

Brand Names	Generic Names	Indications
1. Atrovent		
2. Bentyl		
3. Cogentin		
4. Detrol		
5. Ditropan XL		
6. Donnatal		
7. Enablex		
8. Levsinex		
9. Robinul		
10. Toviaz		
11. Transderm Scōp		
12. VESIcare		

GENERIC NAMES

a. belladonna alkaloids

b. benztropine

c. darifenacin

d. dicyclomine

e. fesoterodine

f. glycopyrrolate

g. hyoscyamine

h. ipratropium

i. oxybutynin

j. scopolamine

k. solifenacin

l. tolterodine

True or False

For additional study, try to change the false statements to make them true.

_____1. Parasympathetic responses are often called cholinergic in reference to the neurotransmitter acetylcholine, the final messenger of this system at the effector organs.

_____2. The PANS is often called the adrenergic nervous system.

_____3. The main types of adrenergic receptors are β1 and α2.

_____4. Anticholinergic and antimuscarinic drugs block the actions of the PANS.

_____5. Epinephrine is a synthetic neurotransmitter that stimulates adrenergic receptors.

_____6. MAO is an enzyme that degrades neurotransmitters in the SANS.

_____7. β agonists can be used to treat bradycardia or asthma.

_____8. β1 antagonists interfere most with the actions of the SANS on the lungs.

Short Answer

1. Why do anticholinergic medications sometimes have actions similar to those that stimulate the sympathetic nervous system?

2. How can pseudoephedrine given for nasal congestion increase a patient's blood pressure?

3. Why are medications that stimulate the SANS sometimes called adrenergic agonists?

4. What are the advantages of using a selective β1 blocker instead of a nonspecific β antagonist in the treatment of hypertension?

5. How do antimuscarinic agents work in the treatment of bladder spasms?

DRUG MONOGRAPH

*Choose one of the agents in **Medication Table 3-3** and complete a drug monograph using the form provided here. (An example of the drug monograph is included in Chapter 1 of this workbook.)*

Generic Name _____

Brand Name _____

Manufacturer _____

APPROVED INDICATION(S)

_____
_____
_____

DOSAGE AND ROUTE(S) OF ADMINISTRATION

_____
_____
_____

AVAILABLE DOSAGE FORM(S) STRENGTH(S)

STORAGE/HANDLING CONDITIONS/PROCEDURES

_____
_____

PRECAUTIONS (CONTRAINDICATIONS, DRUG/FOOD INTERACTIONS, PREGNANCY CATEGORY)

_____
_____
_____
_____

COMMON OR SEVERE ADVERSE REACTIONS

_____
_____
_____
_____
_____

INSTRUCTIONS FOR PATIENTS

_____
_____
_____

COST OF THERAPY (DAILY, MONTHLY, FULL COURSE)

_____
_____

OTHER DRUGS IN THIS CLASS

_____
_____
_____

ADDITIONAL MEDICATIONS WITH SAME INDICATION

_____
_____
_____

ADVANTAGES/DISADVANTAGES COMPARED TO DRUGS LISTED ABOVE (CLASS, INDICATION)

_____
_____
_____
_____

CHAPTER 4

The Central Nervous System

LEARNING OBJECTIVES

After completing this chapter, you should be able to

1. Describe brain and spinal cord anatomy and physiology

2. Define the term neurotransmitter and list functions of each in the central nervous system

3. Identify local and general anesthetics and how each affects the central nervous system

4. Define analgesia and list the effects of opiates and opiate-like medications on the central nervous system

5. List opiate agonists and differentiate their doses, pharmacokinetics, and adverse effects

PRONUNCIATIONS

Analgesia (ann-ul-GEE-zha)
Analgesics (ann-ul-GEE-zikz)
Esterases (ESS-ter-ayss-es)
Glial (GLEE-ul)
Meninges (men-IN-jeez)
Opiate (OH-pee-ut)
Succinylcholine (SUX-i-nil-KOE-leen)
Synapse (SIN-aps)

Matching I

Match each neurotransmitter to a function of the CNS. For additional study, use the space next to the medication to write any abbreviations used for that neurotransmitter.

Neurotransmitters	Functions in CNS	Abbreviations
1. Acetylcholine		
2. Dopamine		
3. Epinephrine		
4. Gamma-amino butyric acid		
5. Glutamate		
6. Histamine		
7. Norepinephrine		
8. Serotonin		

FUNCTIONS OF CNS

a. Activates receptors that deal with memory, reward, and learning

b. Affects attention, movement, and hormone regulation

c. Initiates the "fight-or-flight" response to danger

d. Plays a role in the sleep/wakefulness cycle and in digestion

e. Regulates mood, anger, appetite, sexuality, and body temperature

f. Restrains neuronal circuit activity

g. Stimulates NMDA (receptors)

Matching II

Match each brand name medication to its generic name. Note that some generics are available in more than one brand name. For additional study, use the space next to the medication to mark each drug as an analgesic or anesthetic.

Brand Names	Generic Names	Analgesic/Anesthetic
1. Actiq		
2. Avinza		
3. Demerol		
4. Dilaudid		
5. Diprivan		
6. Duragesic		
7. Kadian		
8. Ketalar		
9. Lidoderm		
10. Marcaine		
11. MS Contin		
12. Novocain		
13. OxyContin		
14. Pontocaine		
15. Roxanol		
16. Sensorcaine		
17. Sublimaze		
18. Ultram		

GENERIC NAMES

a. bupivacaine
b. fentanyl
c. hydromorphone
d. ketamine
e. lidocaine
f. meperidine
g. morphine
h. oxycodone
i. procaine
j. propofol
k. tetracaine
l. tramadol

True or False

For additional study, try to change the false statements to make them true.

_____1. The central nervous system is made up of the brain, spinal cord, SANS, and PANS.

_____2. The neuron is the functional unit of the brain.

_____3. The spinal cord's primary function is to transmit information to and from the brain.

_____4. General anesthetics are applied to a specific part of the body to block the nerves in that part of the body.

_____5. Propofol injections are white and opaque in appearance because they contain milk.

_____6. Local anesthetics for epidural administration must not contain preservatives.

_____7. Two different opioid analgesics are often combined in a single preparation to increase pain relieving potency.

_____8. Potent opioid analgesics are usually classified DEA Schedule II (CII).

_____9. Constipation is a common side effect of opioid analgesics that can often be managed with laxatives or stool softeners.

_____10. Naloxone is a long-acting opiate antagonist used in the management of addiction.

Short Answer

1. What is the blood-brain barrier? How does it work, and how does it affect medication action?

2. Describe the anatomy of a neuron relating each part to its function.

3. Define epidural anesthesia and list some advantages of this route of administration.

4. Describe tolerance, dependence, and addiction and distinguish between and among them.

5. Describe PCA and list some of its advantages.

DRUG MONOGRAPH

Choose one brand name opioid analgesic preparation from **Medication Table 4-1** *and complete a drug monograph, using the form provided here. (An example of the drug monograph is included in Chapter 1 of this workbook.)*

Generic Name _____

Brand Name _____

Manufacturer _____

APPROVED INDICATION(S)

_____
_____
_____
_____

DOSAGE AND ROUTE(S) OF ADMINISTRATION

_____
_____
_____

AVAILABLE DOSAGE FORM(S) STRENGTH(S)

STORAGE/HANDLING CONDITIONS/PROCEDURES

_____
_____
_____

PRECAUTIONS (CONTRAINDICATIONS, DRUG/FOOD INTERACTIONS, PREGNANCY CATEGORY)

_____
_____
_____
_____
_____

COMMON OR SEVERE ADVERSE REACTIONS

_____
_____
_____
_____
_____

INSTRUCTIONS FOR PATIENTS

_____
_____
_____
_____

COST OF THERAPY (DAILY, MONTHLY, FULL COURSE)

_____
_____
_____

OTHER DRUGS IN THIS CLASS

_____
_____
_____

ADDITIONAL MEDICATIONS WITH SAME INDICATION

_____
_____
_____

ADVANTAGES/DISADVANTAGES COMPARED TO DRUGS LISTED ABOVE (CLASS, INDICATION)

_____
_____
_____
_____
_____

CHAPTER 5

Neurologic Disorders

LEARNING OBJECTIVES

After completing this chapter, you should be able to

1. Describe how lesions in the brain and peripheral nervous system are related to neurological diseases

2. List the causes, symptoms, and expected course of the following illnesses:
   - Headache—migraine, cluster, and tension
   - Stroke
   - Parkinson's disease
   - Dementia
   - Epilepsy
   - Multiple sclerosis
   - Neuropathic pain
   - Sleep disorders

3. Describe the psychosocial consequences for patients and families of patients with neurologic disorders

4. State the generic and brand names of medications used to treat neurologic disorders, along with dosage forms and available doses

5. List the mechanism of action, common adverse effects, and special precautions of medications used to treat neurologic disorders

PRONUNCIATIONS

Anticonvulsant (an-tee-kun-VUL-sunt)

Aura (AW-ruh)

Barbiturate (bar-BIT-yur-it)

Benzodiazepine (ben-zoh-die-AZ-uh-peen)

Dementia (di-MEN-shuh)

Neuropathic (nyoor-oh-PATH-ik)

Matching I

Match each disorder to two of its associated symptom(s) listed below.

DISORDERS

_____ _____ 1. Cluster headache

_____ _____ 2. Dementia

_____ _____ 3. Epilepsy

_____ _____ 4. Migraine

_____ _____ 5. Multiple sclerosis

_____ _____ 6. Neuropathic pain

_____ _____ 7. Parkinson's disease

_____ _____ 8. Restless leg syndrome

_____ _____ 9. Sleep apnea

_____ _____ 10. Stroke

ASSOCIATED SYMPTOMS

a. Balance problems

b. Confusion

c. Crawling and/or tingling in legs

d. Loss of consciousness

e. Memory impairment

f. Muscle spasms

g. Numbness and tingling

h. Progressive muscle weakness

i. Seizures

j. Sensitivity to light and/or sound, aura

k. Shooting pains

l. Snoring

m. Stabbing pain of short duration

n. Sudden inability to walk and/or talk

o. Sudden weakness on one side

p. Symptoms relieved by moving the legs

q. Teary eyes and/or runny nose

r. Throbbing on one side of the head

s. Tremor

Matching II

Match each brand name medication to its generic name. For additional study, use the space next to the medication to mark the indication for each drug.

Brand Names	Generic Names	Indications
1. Ambien		
2. Aricept		
3. Artane		
4. Avonex		
5. Azilect		
6. Betaseron		
7. Cerebyx		
8. Cogentin		
9. Cognex		
10. Comtan		
11. Copaxone		
12. Depakote		
13. Dilantin		
14. Dostinex		
15. Exelon		
16. Gabitril		
17. Halcion		
18. Keppra		
19. Klonopin		
20. Lamictal		

Matching III

Match each brand name medication to its generic name. For additional study, use the space next to the medication to mark the indication for each drug.

Brand Names	Generic Names	Indications
1. Lunesta		
2. Lyrica		
3. Mirapex		
4. Mysoline		
5. Namenda		
6. Neurontin		
7. Parlodel		
8. Razadyne		
9. Requip		
10. Restoril		
11. Rozerem		
12. Sinemet		
13. Sonata		
14. Symmetrel		
15. Tasmar		
16. Topamax		
17. Trileptal		
18. Tysabri		
19. Vimpat		
20. Zonegran		

GENERIC NAMES

a. benztropine
b. cabergoline
c. clonazepam
d. divalproex
e. donepezil
f. entacapone
g. fosphenytoin
h. glatiramer
i. interferon beta-1a
j. interferon beta-1b
k. lamotrigine
l. levetiracetam
m. phenytoin
n. rasagiline
o. rivastigmine
p. tacrine
q. tiagabine
r. triazolam
s. trihexyphenidyl
t. zolpidem

GENERIC NAMES

a. amantadine
b. bromocriptine
c. carbidopa/levodopa
d. eszopiclone
e. gabapentin
f. galantamine
g. lacosamide
h. memantine
i. natalizumab
j. oxcarbazepine
k. pramipexole
l. pregabalin
m. primidone
n. ramelteon
o. ropinirole
p. temazepam
q. tolcapone
r. topiramate
s. zaleplon
t. zonisamide

True or False

For additional study, try to change the false statements to make them true.

_____1.   OTC pain medications are always safe for regular use in the treatment of headaches.

_____2.   Migraine headaches can occur in children.

_____3.   A stroke caused by a blood clot in the brain is known as hemorrhagic stroke.

_____4.   Carbidopa is added to PD medications to increase the amount of levodopa that is delivered to the brain.

_____5.   Dementia can be cured by medications such as cholinesterase inhibitors and memantine.

_____6.   The EEG is the most beneficial treatment for epilepsy.

_____7.   Pregabalin and gabapentin are useful only in the treatment of seizures.

_____8.   MS is a disease caused by inflammatory damage to the myelin that normally protects nerve cells.

Short Answer

1.   Describe the recommended approach for the treatment of migraine headache.

2.   How are medications used in the treatment of stroke?

3.   Discuss the side effects that accompany treatments for PD.

4.   Discuss the use of herbals and supplements in the treatment of dementia.

5.   What is meant by good sleep hygiene?

DRUG MONOGRAPH

Choose one brand-name sleep medication from Table 5-6 and complete a drug monograph, using the form provided here. (An example of the drug monograph is included in Chapter 1 of this workbook.)

Generic Name _____

Brand Name _____

Manufacturer _____

APPROVED INDICATION(S)

_____

_____

_____

_____

DOSAGE AND ROUTE(S) OF ADMINISTRATION

_____

_____

_____

AVAILABLE DOSAGE FORM(S) STRENGTH(S)

STORAGE/HANDLING CONDITIONS/PROCEDURES

_____

_____

_____

PRECAUTIONS (CONTRAINDICATIONS, DRUG/FOOD INTERACTIONS, PREGNANCY CATEGORY)

_____

_____

_____

_____

_____

_____

COMMON OR SEVERE ADVERSE REACTIONS

_____

_____

_____

_____

_____

INSTRUCTIONS FOR PATIENTS

_____

_____

_____

_____

COST OF THERAPY (DAILY, MONTHLY, FULL COURSE)

_____

_____

_____

OTHER DRUGS IN THIS CLASS

_____

_____

_____

ADDITIONAL MEDICATIONS WITH SAME INDICATION

_____

_____

_____

_____

ADVANTAGES/DISADVANTAGES COMPARED TO DRUGS LISTED ABOVE (CLASS, INDICATION)

_____

_____

_____

_____

_____

CHAPTER 6

Psychiatric Diseases

LEARNING OBJECTIVES

After completing this chapter, you should be able to

1. Recall what is known of the causes and prevalence of mental illnesses

2. List the symptoms and recall the expected course of the following illnesses:

   • Depression

   • Anxiety disorders

   • Schizophrenia

   • Bipolar disorder

   • Attention deficit hyperactivity disorder

   • Substance abuse

3. Recognize the psychosocial consequences for patients and families of patients with psychiatric disorders

4. State the generic and brand names of medications used to treat psychiatric disorders along with dosage forms and available doses

5. Discuss the mechanism of action, common adverse effects, and special precautions of medications used to treat psychiatric disorders

Matching I

Match each disorder to two of its associated symptom(s) listed below.

DISORDERS

_____ _____1. Anxiety disorders　　_____ _____4. Depression

_____ _____2. ADHD　　　　　　　_____ _____5. Schizophrenia

_____ _____3. Bipolar disorder

ASSOCIATED SYMPTOMS

a. Distractibility

b. Fidgeting

c. Hallucinations

d. Mania

e. Mood fluctuations

f. Obsessive compulsive behavior

g. Paranoia

h. Phobias

i. Sad feelings

j. Suicidal thoughts

PRONUNCIATIONS

Affect (AFF-ekt)

Agoraphobia (ah-GORE-ah-FOE-bee-ah)

Agranulocytosis (AY-gran-yoo-low-sigh-TOE-sis)

Akathesia (AH-kuh-THEEZ-ee-uh)

Antipsychotics (AN-tye-sigh-KOT-iks)

Co-morbidities (koh-more-BID-ih-teez)

Delusion (duh-LOO-zhun)

Dyskinesia (TAR-div-dis-kin-EE-zee-uh)

Dystonia (dis-TOHN-ee-uh)

Enuresis (in-your-EE-sis)

Equipotent (EE-kwi-PO-tent)

Extrapyramidal (EKS-trah-pur-AM-uh-dul)

Hallucination (ha-LOO-sin-AY-shun)

Monoamine oxidase inhibitors (MON-oh-ah-MEEN-OX-i-dase-in-HIB-i-terz)

Pancreatitis (PAN-kree-uh-TY-tis)

Paranoia (PAR-uh-NOY-uh)

Phobia (FOE-be ah)

Prodromal (proe-DROE-mul)

Pseudoparkinsonism (soo-doh-PAR-kin-sun-iz-um)

Psychosis (sie-KO-sis)

Schizophrenia (SKITS-o-FREN-ee-a)

Synapse (SIN-aps)

Matching II

Match each brand name medication to its generic name and classify it as a treatment for ADHD (A) or depression (D). For additional study, use the space to mark the medication class for each drug.

Brand Names	Generic Names	A or D	Medication Class
1. Adderall			
2. Celexa			
3. Concerta			
4. Daytrana			
5. Effexor			
6. Elavil			
7. Intuniv			
8. Lexapro			
9. Pristiq			
10. Prozac			
11. Ritalin			
12. Strattera			
13. Vyvanse			
14. Zoloft			

GENERIC NAMES

a. amitriptyline
b. atomoxetine
c. citalopram
d. desvenlafaxine
e. escitalopram
f. fluoxetine
g. guanfacine
h. lisdexamfetamine
i. methylphenidate
j. mixed amphetamine salts
k. sertraline
l. venlafaxine

Matching III

Match each brand name medication to its generic name. For additional study, use the space to mark the indication for each drug.

Brand Names	Generic Names	Indications
1. Abilify		
2. Antabuse		
3. Ativan		
4. Campral		
5. Chantix		
6. Clozaril		
7. Haldol		
8. Nicoderm		
9. Nicorette		
10. Prolixin		
11. Risperdal		
12. Suboxone		
13. Valium		
14. Xanax		
15. Zyban		
16. Zyprexa		

GENERIC NAMES

a. acamprosate
b. alprazolam
c. aripiprazole
d. buprenorphine/naloxone
e. bupropion
f. clozapine
g. diazepam
h. disulfiram
i. fluphenazine
j. haloperidol
k. lorazepam
l. nicotine
m. olanzapine
n. risperidone
o. varenicline

True or False

For additional study, try to change the false statements to make them true.

_____1. Psychiatric disorders are usually detected in the results from blood testing.

_____2. Symptoms of depression vary from patient to patient.

_____3. Antidepressants do not act immediately and usually must be taken for weeks before an effect is seen.

_____4. Patients taking benzodiazepines for anxiety need not be concerned about side effects.

_____5. Schizophrenia can usually be cured by appropriate medication therapy.

_____6. Atypical antipsychotics may cause weight gain, diabetes, and cardiovascular side effects.

_____7. Bipolar disorder is often treated with drugs that are also used for epilepsy.

_____8. Lithium is the oldest and best studied medication for ADHD.

_____9. Most children diagnosed with ADHD will out grow the disease by adulthood.

_____10. Addiction and dependence are two words that mean essentially the same thing.

Short Answer

1. List some ways in which psychiatric disorders must be diagnosed and treated differently from other medical conditions.

2. Name the major classes of antidepressants and give an example of each. What feature do all have in common?

3. Name some benzodiazepines used to treat anxiety including at least one short-acting and one longer acting agent. Which other drugs in this class are used to treat insomnia?

4. Name two classes of antipsychotic drugs with examples of each. Give some of the major side effects.

5. Name at least two mood stabilizers used to treat bipolar disorder. Are they used for any other condition?

DRUG MONOGRAPH

*Choose one brand-name ADHD medication from **Medication Table 6-4** and complete a drug monograph using the form provided here. (An example of the drug monograph is included in Chapter 1 of this workbook.)*

Generic Name _____

Brand Name _____

Manufacturer _____

APPROVED INDICATION(S)

_____
_____
_____
_____

DOSAGE AND ROUTE(S) OF ADMINISTRATION

_____
_____
_____

AVAILABLE DOSAGE FORM(S) STRENGTH(S)

STORAGE/HANDLING CONDITIONS/PROCEDURES

_____
_____

PRECAUTIONS (CONTRAINDICATIONS, DRUG/FOOD INTERACTIONS, PREGNANCY CATEGORY)

_____
_____
_____
_____
_____

COMMON OR SEVERE ADVERSE REACTIONS

_____
_____
_____
_____
_____

INSTRUCTIONS FOR PATIENTS

_____
_____
_____
_____

COST OF THERAPY (DAILY, MONTHLY, FULL COURSE)

_____
_____
_____

OTHER DRUGS IN THIS CLASS

_____
_____
_____

ADDITIONAL MEDICATIONS WITH SAME INDICATION

_____
_____
_____
_____

ADVANTAGES/DISADVANTAGES COMPARED TO DRUGS LISTED ABOVE (CLASS, INDICATION)

_____
_____
_____
_____
_____

CHAPTER 7

Overview of the Endocrine System and Agents

LEARNING OBJECTIVES

After completing this chapter, you should be able to

1. Describe the negative feedback system used to regulate levels of many of the body's hormones

2. Define the following:
   - Acromegaly
   - Hyperparathyroidism
   - Hyperthyroidism
   - Hypoparathyroidism
   - Hypopituitarism
   - Hypothyroidism

3. State the brand and generic names of the most widely prescribed medications for pituitary disorders, thyroid disorders, and parathyroid disorders

4. Be familiar with their routes of administration and dosage forms, and the most common adverse effects of medications used to treat pituitary disorders, thyroid disorders, and parathyroid disorders

5. Describe the therapeutic effects of medications used to treat pituitary disorders, thyroid disorders, and parathyroid disorders

Matching I

Match each disorder to its symptoms and treatment.

Disorders	Symptoms	Treatments
Acromegaly		
Hyperparathyroidism		
Hyperthyroidism		
Hypothyroidism		

SYMPTOMS

a. Heart disease, hypertension, osteoarthritis
b. Osteodystrophy, vitamin D deficiency
c. Weight gain, fatigue, dry skin, depression
d. Weight loss, sweating, nervousness, insomnia

TREATMENT

1. Levothyroxine, liothyronine, liotrix
2. Octreotide, bromocriptine, cabergoline
3. Propylthiouracil, methimazole
4. Sevelamer, aluminum carbonate

Matching II

Match each brand name to its generic name. For additional study, use the space to write the condition for which the drug is used.

Brand Names	Generic Names	Conditions
1. Forteo		
2. Levoxyl		
3. Miacalcin		
4. Parlodel		
5. PhosLo		
6. Renagel		
7. Rocaltrol		
8. Sandostatin		
9. Synthroid		

GENERIC NAMES

a. bromocriptine   e. levothyroxine

b. calcitonin salmon   f. octreotide

c. calcitriol   g. sevelamer

d. calcium acetate   h. teriparatide

True or False

For additional study, try to change the false statements to make them true.

_____1. The primary function of hormones is to regulate sexual desires and characteristics.

_____2. The thyroid gland has two lobes and is located in the brain.

_____3. Hypothyroid patients whose dosage of levothyroxine is too high may experience symptoms of hyperthyroidism.

_____4. The only relationship between the thyroid and parathyroid glands is their location near one another in the neck.

_____5. A condition caused by growth hormone (GH) deficiency is acromegaly.

_____6. Octreotide is available as an oral preparation taken every 5 weeks to control GH levels.

_____7. Hyperthyroidism is treated with liothyronine or liotrix.

_____8. Parathyroid hormone (PTH) regulates calcium concentrations in the blood.

_____9. Calcitriol is a synthetic PTH replacement.

_____10. Patients with chronic kidney disease often require vitamin D therapy with active forms of the vitamin such as paricalcitol or calcitriol.

Short Answer

1. Name the pituitary hormones and their functions.

2. Name the thyroid hormones and their functions.

3. What hormone is produced by the parathyroid, and what does it do?

4. What medications are prescribed for patients with chronic kidney disease who have secondary hyperparathyroidism? Why?

5. Name some of the available vitamin D preparations. Which can be administered orally?

DRUG MONOGRAPH

*Choose one brand-name thyroid supplement from **Medication Table 7-2** and complete a drug monograph using the form provided here. (An example of the drug monograph is included in Chapter 1 of this workbook.)*

Generic Name _____

Brand Name _____

Manufacturer _____

APPROVED INDICATION(S)

_____

_____

_____

_____

DOSAGE AND ROUTE(S) OF ADMINISTRATION

_____

_____

_____

AVAILABLE DOSAGE FORM(S) STRENGTH(S)

STORAGE/HANDLING CONDITIONS/PROCEDURES

_____

_____

_____

PRECAUTIONS (CONTRAINDICATIONS, DRUG/FOOD INTERACTIONS, PREGNANCY CATEGORY)

_____

_____

_____

_____

_____

_____

COMMON OR SEVERE ADVERSE REACTIONS

_____

_____

_____

_____

INSTRUCTIONS FOR PATIENTS

_____

_____

_____

_____

COST OF THERAPY (DAILY, MONTHLY, FULL COURSE)

_____

_____

_____

OTHER DRUGS IN THIS CLASS

_____

_____

_____

ADDITIONAL MEDICATIONS WITH SAME INDICATION

_____

_____

_____

_____

ADVANTAGES/DISADVANTAGES COMPARED TO DRUGS LISTED ABOVE (CLASS, INDICATION)

_____

_____

_____

_____

_____

CHAPTER 8

Adrenal Gland Hormones

LEARNING OBJECTIVES

After completing this chapter, you should be able to

1. Identify the hormones produced by the adrenal glands
2. Describe the functions of mineralocorticoids and glucocorticoids in the body
3. Recognize the signs and symptoms of adrenal insufficiency
4. Describe the pharmacological treatment of patients with acute and chronic adrenal insufficiency
5. Recognize the signs and symptoms of Cushing's syndrome and the result of too much cortisol
6. Describe the pharmacologic and nonpharmacologic management of patients with Cushing's syndrome
7. List management strategies for administration of glucocorticoid and mineralocorticoid therapy to avoid development of adrenal disorders

PRONUNCIATIONS

Adrenocorticotropic (ad-RENE-no-CORE-ti-co-TRO-pic)

Aldosterone (al-DOS-te-rone)

Corticotropin (CORE-ti-co-TRO-pin)

Cortisol (CORE-ti-sol)

Glucocorticoids (glu-co-CORE-ti-coids)

Hypercortisolism (hy-per-CORE-ti-SOLE-ism)

Hyperpigmentation (hi-per-pig-men-TAY-tion)

Hypocortisolism (hy-po-CORE-ti-sol-ism)

Hypothalamus (hy-po-THAL-a-mus)

Mineralocorticoids (min-er-al-o-CORE-ti-coids)

Pituitary (PIT-tu-IT-tary)

Steroidogenesis (ste-ROID-o-JEN-eh-sis)

Matching I

Identify the endogenous adrenal hormone associated with each physiologic action. For additional study, name an exogenous hormone medication that accomplishes this action.

Actions	Hormones	Exogenous Hormone Medication
Anti-inflammatory effect		
Immune response suppression		
Potassium depletion		
Regulation of blood glucose		
Sexual maturation		
Sodium retention		
Water retention		

HORMONES

a. Aldosterone (mineralocorticoid)
b. Androgen
c. Cortisol (glucocorticoid)

Matching II

Match each brand name to its generic name. For additional study, use the space to write the route of administration for each preparation.

Brand Names	Generic Names	Route of Administration
1. Cortaid		
2. Cortef		
3. Cortifoam		
4. Depo-Medrol		
5. Diprolene		
6. Elocon		
7. Kenalog		
8. Medrol		
9. Solu-Cortef		
10. Solu-Medrol		
11. Synalar		
12. Topicort		

GENERIC NAMES

a. betamethasone
b. desoximetasone
c. fluocinolone
d. hydrocortisone
e. methylprednisolone
f. mometasone
g. triamcinolone

True or False

For additional study, try to change the false statements to make them true.

_____1. The adrenal medulla secretes the hormone neurotransmitters epinephrine and norepinephrine.

_____2. ACTH secreted by the adrenal gland stimulates the pituitary gland.

_____3. Hydrocortisone is the primary glucocorticoid secreted by the adrenal glands.

_____4. Aldosterone is the primary mineralocorticoid secreted by the adrenal glands.

_____5. The glucocorticoid medications are called steroids and have been used to build muscle mass and athletic performance.

_____6. Glucocorticoids are useful in the treatment of inflammatory conditions such as arthritis.

_____7. Allergic reactions are common side effects of dermatologic corticosteroids.

_____8. Hydrocortisone cream is available over-the-counter.

_____9. Hydrocortisone oral tablets are available over-the-counter.

_____10. Increases in blood sugar are associated with long-term corticosteroid therapy.

Short Answer

1. Describe the position and anatomy of the adrenal glands.

2. List some indications for administration of exogenous glucocorticoid medications.

3. Which corticosteroid medications have the highest ratio of glucocorticoid to mineralocorticoid activity? What is the significance of this?

4. What is Cushing's syndrome? How is it treated?

5. When patients receive supplemental corticosteroid doses to prevent adrenal crisis, what is the proper way to revert to their normal dose once the crisis has passed?

DRUG MONOGRAPH

*Choose one brand-name systemic corticosteroid preparation from **Medication Table 8-2** and complete a drug monograph using the form provided here. (An example of the drug monograph is included in Chapter 1 of this workbook.)*

Generic Name _____

Brand Name _____

Manufacturer _____

APPROVED INDICATION(S)

_____
_____
_____
_____

DOSAGE AND ROUTE(S) OF ADMINISTRATION

_____
_____
_____
_____

AVAILABLE DOSAGE FORM(S) STRENGTH(S)

STORAGE/HANDLING CONDITIONS/PROCEDURES

_____
_____
_____

PRECAUTIONS (CONTRAINDICATIONS, DRUG/FOOD INTERACTIONS, PREGNANCY CATEGORY)

_____
_____
_____
_____
_____

COMMON OR SEVERE ADVERSE REACTIONS

_____
_____
_____
_____
_____

INSTRUCTIONS FOR PATIENTS

_____
_____
_____
_____
_____

COST OF THERAPY (DAILY, MONTHLY, FULL COURSE)

_____
_____
_____

OTHER DRUGS IN THIS CLASS

_____
_____
_____

ADDITIONAL MEDICATIONS WITH SAME INDICATION

_____
_____
_____
_____

ADVANTAGES/DISADVANTAGES COMPARED TO DRUGS LISTED ABOVE (CLASS, INDICATION)

_____
_____
_____
_____
_____

CHAPTER 9

Diabetes

LEARNING OBJECTIVES

After completing this chapter, you should be able to

1. Define the following:
   - Diabetes mellitus, type 1 and type 2
   - Metabolic syndrome
   - Glycosylated hemoglobin (HbA$_{1c}$)

2. Outline the physiology of normal carbohydrate metabolism and the role of pancreatic hormones

3. List the causes and results of diabetes mellitus and metabolic syndrome

4. Describe nonpharmacologic therapies for diabetes mellitus

5. Review the therapeutic effects of insulin and oral hypoglycemic medications and list their most common side effects and adverse reactions

6. State the brand and generic names of the most widely used hypoglycemic medications, along with their routes of administration, dosage forms, and available doses

7. Recognize common regimens for the treatment of diabetes mellitus

PRONUNCIATIONS

Alpha-Glucosidase (AL-fa-glue-COSS-i-dace)

Biguanides (bie-GWON-ides)

Diabetes mellitus (die-a-BEET-es MEL-et-us)

Glycemic (glie-SEE-mic)

Glycosylated hemoglobin (glie-KOS-il-ay-ted HEE-muh-gloe-bin)

Ketoacidosis (kee-toe-ass-i-DOE-sis)

Lipoatrophy (lip-oh-AT-roh-fee)

Lipodystrophy (lip-oh-DISS-troh-fee)

Lipohypertrophy (lip-oh-hie-PER-troh-fee)

Meglitinides (me-GLIT-in-ides)

Secretagogue (si-KREE-ta-gog)

Sulfonylureas (sul-fon-il-YOR-ee-as)

Thiazolidinedione (thie-a-zoe-li-deen-DIE-oen)

Matching I

Match the brand name to its generic equivalent for each insulin product, and identify its duration of action as **R** *(rapid),* **S** *(short),* **I** *(intermediate), or* **L** *(long).*

Brand Names	Generic Names	Duration of Action
1. Apidra		
2. Humalog		
3. Humulin N		
4. Humulin R		
5. Lantus		
6. Levemir		
7. Novolin N		
8. Novolin R		
9. NovoLog		

GENERIC NAMES

a. insulin aspart

b. insulin detemir

c. insulin glargine

d. insulin glulisine

e. insulin lispro

f. isophane (NPH) insulin

g. regular human insulin

Matching II

Match each brand name to its generic name and list its route of administration. For addtional study, use the space to write each drug's mechanism of action.

Brand Names	Generic Names	Routes	Mechanism of Action
1. Actos			
2. Avandia			
3. Byetta			
4. Glucophage			
5. Glucotrol			
6. Januvia			
7. Prandin			
8. Starlix			
9. Symlin			
10. Tradjenta			

GENERIC NAMES

a. exenatide   f. pioglitazone

b. glipizide   g. pramlintide

c. linagliptin   h. repaglinide

d. metformin   i. rosiglitazone

e. nateglinide   j. sitagliptin

True or False

For additional study, try to change the false statements to make them true.

_____1. All diabetes is related to a reduced sensitivity of the body's cells to the actions of insulin.

_____2. Complications of diabetes are serious, but not life-threatening.

_____3. Hyperglycemia is a blood glucose level that is higher than normal.

_____4. Insulin injections should be always be administered to the same place to promote consistency in absorption.

_____5. Many patients with Type 2 diabetes can be treated with oral medications that would not be useful for patients with Type 1.

_____6. Alpha-glucosidase inhibitors such as acarbose should be taken on an empty stomach.

_____7. Many patients require a combination of medications with different mechanisms of action to achieve their glycemic goals.

_____8. Metformin acts on the beta cells in the pancreas to increase insulin production.

_____9. Sitagliptin has been associated with an increased risk of myocardial infarction and cardiac death.

_____10. Insulins must be injected, but other therapies for diabetes can all be administered orally.

Short Answer

1. Describe metabolic syndrome and the health risks for patients who have this disorder.

2. Why must patients with Type 1 diabetes be treated with insulin while some patients with Type 2 can get by without it?

3. Why is insulin administered by injection (or perhaps inhalation) and not by mouth the way some other medications for diabetes are?

4. What is SMBG, and why do diabetic patients use it?

5. What side effect is most common among medications used to treat diabetes?

DRUG MONOGRAPH

*Choose one brand-name oral preparation from **Medication Table 9-2** and complete a drug monograph using the form provided here. (An example of the drug monograph is included in Chapter 1 of this workbook.)*

Generic Name _____

Brand Name _____

Manufacturer _____

APPROVED INDICATION(S)

_____
_____
_____
_____

DOSAGE AND ROUTE(S) OF ADMINISTRATION

_____
_____
_____

AVAILABLE DOSAGE FORM(S) STRENGTH(S)

STORAGE/HANDLING CONDITIONS/PROCEDURES

_____
_____
_____

PRECAUTIONS (CONTRAINDICATIONS, DRUG/FOOD INTERACTIONS, PREGNANCY CATEGORY)

_____
_____
_____
_____
_____

COMMON OR SEVERE ADVERSE REACTIONS

_____
_____
_____
_____
_____
_____

INSTRUCTIONS FOR PATIENTS

_____
_____
_____
_____

COST OF THERAPY (DAILY, MONTHLY, FULL COURSE)

_____
_____
_____

OTHER DRUGS IN THIS CLASS

_____
_____
_____

ADDITIONAL MEDICATIONS WITH SAME INDICATION

_____
_____
_____

ADVANTAGES/DISADVANTAGES COMPARED TO DRUGS LISTED ABOVE (CLASS, INDICATION)

_____
_____
_____
_____
_____

CHAPTER 10

Reproductive Hormones

LEARNING OBJECTIVES

After completing this chapter, you should be able to

1. List the physiologic roles for each of the major reproductive hormones

2. Recognize common therapeutic indications for the use of reproductive hormones

3. Recognize available dosage forms and describe adverse effects, administration, storage, and handling techniques for the available estrogen and progestin preparations

4. Recognize available dosage forms and describe adverse effects, administration, storage, and handling techniques for the available testosterone preparations

5. Recognize available dosage forms and describe adverse effects, administration, storage, and handling techniques for the available preparations to treat benign prostatic hyperplasia

Matching I

Match each hormone to the function it serves in the body and the organ that secretes it. For additional study, write out the full names of the abbreviated hormones.

Hormones	Functions	Gland/Organ	Full Name
1. Estrogen			
2. FSH			
3. GnRH			
4. LH			
5. Progesterone			
6. Testosterone			

FUNCTIONS

a. Maintains ovulation cycle

b. Primary female sex hormone

c. Primary male sex hormone

d. Promotes sperm and egg maturation

e. Stimulates release of primary sex hormones

f. Stimulates secretion of LH

GLAND/ORGAN

H. Hypothalamus

O. Ovary

P. Pituitary

T. Testicle

PRONUNCIATIONS

Amenorrhea (ay-MEN-or-EE-ah)

Androgenic (an-dro-JEN-ic)

Aromatase (air-OH-ma-tase)

Atrophic vaginitis (aa-TROH-fic vaa-jin-EYE-tis)

Chorionic (cory-ON-ic)

Dihydrotestosterone (DI-hy-dro-tes-TOS-te-rone)

Dysmenorrhea (DISS-men-or-EE-ah)

Dyspareunia (dis-pair-OO-nee-ah)

Endometrial (endo-MEE-tree-al)

Endometrial hyperplasia (en-doh-MEE-tree-ul hie-per-PLAY-zha)

Endometriosis (EN-doe-MEE-tree-OH-sis)

Endometrium (en-doe-MEE-tree-um)

Estrogenic (es-tro-JEN-ic)

Exogenous (ex-AH-jen-us)

Gonadotropins (go-NAD-oh-TROW-pins)

Gynecomastia (GYE-nuh-coh-MAST-ee-uh)

Hirsutism (her-SOO-tism)

Hypogonadism (hye-poe-GOE-nad-izm)

Luteinizing (LOO-ten-EYE-zing)

Menorrhagia (men-or-RAH-zjuh)

Menses (MEN-seez)

Ovarian (oh-VAIR-ee-un)

Progestogenic (pro-JESS-toe-JEN-ic)

Reductase (re-DUCK-tase)

Vasomotor (VAYZ-oh-MOW-ter)

Yuzpe (YOOZ-pee)

Matching II

Match each brand name to its generic name and its indication.

Brand Names	Generic Names	Indications
1. Androderm		
2. AndroGel		
3. Angeliq		
4. Avodart		
5. Casodex		
6. Depo-Provera		
7. Flomax		
8. Gianvi		
9. Loestrin 24 FE		
10. Lupron		
11. NuvaRing		
12. Ocella		
13. Premarin		
14. Prempro		
15. Proscar		
16. Provera		
17. TriNessa-28		
18. Tri-Sprintec		
19. Vivelle		
20. Yaz		

GENERIC NAMES

a. bicalutamide

b. conjugated estrogens

c. conjugated estrogens+ medroxyprogesterone

d. dutasteride

e. ethinyl estradiol+ etonogestrel

f. ethinyl estradiol+ drospirenone

g. ethinyl estradiol+ norethindrone+iron

h. ethinyl estradiol+ norgestimate

i. estradiol + drospirenone

j. estradiol transdermal

k. finasteride

l. leuprolide

m. medroxyprogesterone

n. tamsulosin

o. testosterone transdermal

INDICATIONS

• BPH

• Contraception

• Female hormone replacement

• Male hormone replacement

• Prostate cancer

True or False

For additional study, try to change the false statements to make them true.

_____1. Menopause is the period of a woman's life when menstruation occurs and a pregnancy can be maintained.

_____2. Estrogens are sex hormones, but they also have effects on bone health, blood clotting, and cholesterol.

_____3. Preparations that combine estrogen and progesterone are used for contraception, reduction of menstrual symptoms, and treatment of acne.

_____4. A four-phasic contraceptive regimen is defined as one that reduces the frequency of menses to four times per year.

_____5. All hormonal contraceptive regimens are administered orally.

_____6. Emergency contraception such as Plan B is available only by prescription and must be started within 12 hours of unprotected intercourse.

_____7. Treatment of menopausal issues focuses on symptomatic relief, improvement in quality of life, and minimizing the risk of side effects and complications relating to therapy.

_____8. Estrogen therapy for the treatment of menopause symptoms is FDA-approved.

_____9. Although convenient, transdermal and intravaginal estrogen treatment is more likely to result in side effects than oral therapy.

_____10. Androgen receptor blockers decrease the effects of testosterone and may be used to treat prostate cancer.

Short Answer

1. Describe common side effects of combined oral contraceptives. What serious adverse reactions have been associated with them?

2. Describe the information included in the medication guide and patient leaflets dispensed with hormonal contraception.

4. What is the indication for clomiphene citrate? How does it work, and what side effects are associated with it?

3. Describe the Yuzpe method of emergency contraception.

5. What is BPH? What two classes of drugs are most often used to treat it?

DRUG MONOGRAPH

Choose one brand-name testosterone replacement product and complete a drug monograph using the form provided here. (An example of the drug monograph is included in Chapter 1 of this workbook.)

Generic Name _____

Brand Name _____

Manufacturer _____

APPROVED INDICATION(S)

_____
_____
_____
_____

DOSAGE AND ROUTE(S) OF ADMINISTRATION

_____
_____
_____

AVAILABLE DOSAGE FORM(S) STRENGTH(S)

STORAGE/HANDLING CONDITIONS/PROCEDURES

_____
_____
_____

PRECAUTIONS (CONTRAINDICATIONS, DRUG/FOOD INTERACTIONS, PREGNANCY CATEGORY)

_____
_____
_____
_____
_____

COMMON OR SEVERE ADVERSE REACTIONS

_____
_____
_____
_____
_____

INSTRUCTIONS FOR PATIENTS

_____
_____
_____
_____

COST OF THERAPY (DAILY, MONTHLY, FULL COURSE)

_____
_____
_____

OTHER DRUGS IN THIS CLASS

_____
_____
_____

ADDITIONAL MEDICATIONS WITH SAME INDICATION

_____
_____
_____

ADVANTAGES/DISADVANTAGES COMPARED TO DRUGS LISTED ABOVE (CLASS, INDICATION)

_____
_____
_____
_____
_____

CHAPTER 11

Overview of the Musculoskeletal System

LEARNING OBJECTIVES

After completing this chapter, you should be able to

1. Describe the basic anatomy and physiology of the musculoskeletal system and its relationship to the central and peripheral nervous systems

2. List common conditions causing musculoskeletal pain

3. Discuss the different categories of skeletal muscle relaxants and state their common uses

4. Recognize neuromuscular blocking agents used in surgery or procedures

5. State the generic names of widely used skeletal muscle relaxants used to treat muscle pain in the acute setting

6. List the general mechanisms of action, therapeutic benefit, and adverse effects of some of the most common skeletal muscle relaxants

PRONUNCIATIONS

Antispasmodics (an-tye-spaz-MOD-iks)

Spasmolytic (spaz-moh-LIT-ik)

Matching I

Match the brand name to its generic equivalent and indicate whether it is a skeletal muscle relaxant (S) or a neuromuscular blocking agent (N). For additional study, note which ones are available as injections.

Brand Names	Generic Names	Class (S or N)	Injectable Available?
1. Anectine			
2. Dantrium			
3. Flexeril			
4. Lioresal			
5. Nimbex			
6. Norflex			
7. Parafon Forte			
8. Quelicin			
9. Robaxin			
10. Skelaxin			
11. Soma Compound			
12. Soma			
13. Zanaflex			
14. Zemuron			

GENERIC NAMES

a. baclofen
b. carisoprodol
c. carisoprodol/aspirin
d. chlorzoxazone
e. cisatracurium

f. cyclobenzaprine
g. dantrolene
h. metaxolone
i. methocarbamol

j. orphenadrine
k. rocuronium
l. succinylcholine
m. tizanidine

Matching II

Match each medication to its associated side or adverse effect.

Medications	Side/Adverse Effects
1. atracurium	
2. chlorzoxazone	
3. cisatracurium	
4. cyclobenzaprine	
5. methocarbamol	
6. orphenadrine	
7. succinylcholine	
8. tizanidine	

SIDE/ADVERSE EFFECTS

a. Apnea

b. Drowsiness

c. Flushing

d. Hypotension

e. Malignant hypothermia

f. Urine discoloration

True or False

For additional study, try to change the false statements to make them true.

_____1. Musculoskeletal pain is a rare but life-threatening condition.

_____2. Muscle pain can result when muscles are injured or underused.

_____3. The first-line treatment for muscle strain is a skeletal muscle relaxant.

_____4. Neuromuscular blocking agents are usually prescribed to treat chronic conditions causing generalized muscle cramping, increased muscle tone, or spasticity.

_____5. It is not unusual for patients to be taking both spasmolytics and pain relievers together for muscle injuries.

_____6. Bed rest is the recommended treatment of acute low back pain related to a muscle strain.

_____7. Intravenous dantrolene should be reconstituted in advance of need because it is an emergency drug for a life-threatening condition.

_____8. Baclofen injection can be administered directly into the spinal fluid for treatment of spastic conditions.

_____9. Succinylcholine is a long-acting neuromuscular blocking agent.

_____10. Nondepolarizing neuromuscular blocking agents are relatively safe and free of adverse effects.

Short Answer

1. Discuss the differences and similarities between sprains and strains, including their causes and symptoms.

2. What is the rationale for using spasmolytics to treat back pain caused by muscle strain?

3. What are some common side effects of centrally-acting spasmolytics, and what warnings should patients receive because of them?

4. What chronic conditions may be treated with antispasmodics?

5. Why is it sometimes desirable to administer an ultra-short-acting neuromuscular blocker but sometimes better to use a longer acting agent?

DRUG MONOGRAPH

*Choose one brand-name muscle relaxant from the **Medication Tables** in Chapter 11 and complete a drug monograph using the form provided here. (An example of the drug monograph is included in Chapter 1 of this workbook.)*

Generic Name _____

Brand Name _____

Manufacturer _____

APPROVED INDICATION(S)

_____
_____
_____
_____

DOSAGE AND ROUTE(S) OF ADMINISTRATION

_____
_____
_____

AVAILABLE DOSAGE FORM(S) STRENGTH(S)

STORAGE/HANDLING CONDITIONS/PROCEDURES

_____
_____
_____

PRECAUTIONS (CONTRAINDICATIONS, DRUG/FOOD INTERACTIONS, PREGNANCY CATEGORY)

_____
_____
_____
_____
_____

COMMON OR SEVERE ADVERSE REACTIONS

_____
_____
_____
_____
_____
_____

INSTRUCTIONS FOR PATIENTS

_____
_____
_____
_____

COST OF THERAPY (DAILY, MONTHLY, FULL COURSE)

_____
_____
_____

OTHER DRUGS IN THIS CLASS

_____
_____

ADDITIONAL MEDICATIONS WITH SAME INDICATION

_____
_____
_____
_____

ADVANTAGES/DISADVANTAGES COMPARED TO DRUGS LISTED ABOVE (CLASS, INDICATION)

_____
_____
_____
_____
_____

PART 4

CHAPTER 12

Musculoskeletal Disorders

LEARNING OBJECTIVES

After completing this chapter, you should be able to

1. Recognize the cause of gouty arthritis and list the therapies to prevent an attack

2. Describe prescription and supplemental therapies for osteoporosis

3. Calculate the amount of elemental calcium in a calcium supplement

4. Describe prescription and supplemental therapies for osteoarthritis

5. Recognize common regimens for rheumatoid arthritis and their adverse effects

6. Recognize common symptoms of and organs affected by systemic lupus erythematosus

7. State the brand and generic names of widely used medications for musculo-skeletal conditions along with their routes of administrations and dosage forms available

PRONUNCIATIONS

Bisphosphonates (bye-FOS-foh-nate)

Corticosteroids (kor-tuh-koh-STAIR-oid)

Cytokines (SIE-toh-kines)

Hyaluronan (hi-al-YER-ah-nan)

Necrosis (ne-KROH-sis)

Osteoarthritis (ahs-tee-oh-ahr-THRY-tis)

Osteomalacia (ahs-tee-oh-muh-LAY-shuh)

Osteonecrosis (ahs-tee-oh-neh-KROH-sis)

Osteoporosis (ahs-tee-oh-por-OH-sis)

Raynaud's (RAY-nodz) phenom-enon

Rheumatoid (ROO-muh-toid)

Matching I

Match each condition to its symptoms. For additional study, write the cause next to the symptoms.

Conditions	Symptoms	Cause
1. Gouty arthritis		
2. Osteoarthritis		
3. Osteoporosis		
4. Rheumatoid arthritis		
5. Systemic lupus erythematosus		

SYMPTOMS

a. Brittle bones (bones that break easily)

b. Joint pain in great toe

c. Joint pain, butterfly rash, fatigue

d. Joint pain, morning stiffness

e. Symmetrical joint pain, all-day stiffness

Matching II

Match each brand name to its generic name and indication(s). For additional study, use the space to write each route of administration.

Brand Names	Generic Names	Indica-tion	Route of Administration
1. Actonel			
2. Boniva			
3. Colcrys			
4. Enbrel			
5. Forteo			
6. Fortical			
7. Fosamax			
8. Humira			
9. Krystexxa			
10. Miacalcin			
11. Plaquenil			
12. Remicade			
13. Rheuma-trex			
14. Uloric			
15. Zyloprim			

GENERIC NAMES

a. adalimumab
b. alendronate
c. allopurinol
d. calcitonin
e. colchicine
f. etanercept
g. febuxostat
h. hydroxychloroquine
i. ibandronate
j. infliximab
k. methotrexate
l. pegloticase
m. risedronate
n. teriparatide

INDICATIONS

O = Osteoporosis
R = Rheumatoid arthritis
T = Gout

Matching III

Match each brand name to its generic name. For additional study, mark the medications that are considered NSAIDs.

Brand Names	Generic Names	NSAIDs
1. Advil		
2. Aleve		
3. Celebrex		
4. Dolobid		
5. Flector		
6. Motrin		
7. Rybix		
8. Tylenol		
9. Ultram		
10. Voltaren		

GENERIC NAMES

a. acetaminophen
b. celecoxib
c. diclofenac
d. diflunisal
e. ibuprofen
f. naproxen
g. tramadol

True or False

For additional study, try to change the false statements to make them true.

_____1. Osteoarthritis, gout, and osteoporosis are common conditions frequently treated with medications.

_____2. High uric acid levels usually lead to gout attacks so they should be treated proactively with medication.

_____3. Pegloticase is a convenient treatment for home use because it is needed only every two weeks.

_____4. Although women are at highest risk for osteoporosis, men can also be diagnosed with this condition.

_____5. Oral bisphosphonates for osteoporosis are well absorbed and can be taken without regard to mealtimes.

_____6. Rheumatoid arthritis and osteoarthritis both cause pain and stiffness in the joints.

_____7. Osteoarthritis is treated with corticosteroids, NSAIDs, and DMARDs.

_____8. Even the NSAIDs that are available in OTC dosage forms can have serious or life-threatening side effects.

_____9.	Unlike conventional DMARDs, biologic DMARDs are relatively free of serious side effects.

_____10.	The primary therapy for treatment of SLE is a regimen of medications to suppress the immune system to prevent it from attacking body tissues.

Short Answer

1.	Describe the mechanism of action for medications used to prevent gout attacks.

2.	Explain why vitamin D is often included as part of calcium supplementation for osteoporosis.

3.	What nutritional supplements, in what doses, are sometimes recommended for osteoarthritis? Why are they not part of the standard therapy for this condition?

4.	What is represented by the acronym DMARD? What is the mechanism of action of this type of agent in the treatment of rheumatoid arthritis?

5.	What organ systems can be affected by SLE?

DRUG MONOGRAPH

*Choose one brand-name tumor necrosis factor (TNF) blocker from **Table 12-5** and complete a drug monograph, using the form provided here. (An example of the drug monograph is included in Chapter 1 of this workbook.)*

Generic Name _____

Brand Name _____

Manufacturer _____

APPROVED INDICATION(S)

_____
_____
_____
_____

DOSAGE AND ROUTE(S) OF ADMINISTRATION

_____
_____
_____

AVAILABLE DOSAGE FORM(S) STRENGTH(S)

STORAGE/HANDLING CONDITIONS/PROCEDURES

_____
_____
_____

PRECAUTIONS (CONTRAINDICATIONS, DRUG/FOOD INTERACTIONS, PREGNANCY CATEGORY)

_____
_____
_____
_____
_____

COMMON OR SEVERE ADVERSE REACTIONS

_____
_____
_____
_____
_____

INSTRUCTIONS FOR PATIENTS

_____
_____
_____
_____

COST OF THERAPY (DAILY, MONTHLY, FULL COURSE)

_____
_____

OTHER DRUGS IN THIS CLASS

_____
_____
_____

ADDITIONAL MEDICATIONS WITH SAME INDICATION

_____
_____
_____

ADVANTAGES/DISADVANTAGES COMPARED TO DRUGS LISTED ABOVE (CLASS, INDICATION)

_____
_____
_____
_____

CHAPTER 13

Overview of the Cardiovascular and Renal Systems

LEARNING OBJECTIVES

After completing this chapter, you should be able to

1. Describe the structure of the heart, including the chambers, valves, and conduction systems
2. Review the course of blood flow around the body from the arterial system to capillaries to the venous system
3. Describe the gross anatomy of the kidney and its functional unit, the nephron
4. List the major classes of diuretics and their sites of action in the nephron
5. Explain the pathophysiology of kidney stones, diabetes insipidus, and nephropathy and the common strategies used to treat them

Matching I

Match each label to the part of the heart or kidney it represents. For additional study, write the function of the structure next to the label. Use the table below.

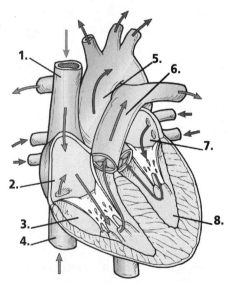

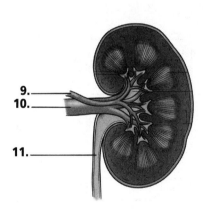

Label	#	Function	Label	#	Function
a. Aorta			g. Renal vein		
b. Inferior vena cava			h. Right atrium		
c. Left atrium			i. Right ventricle		
d. Left ventricle			j. Superior vena cava		
e. Pulmonary artery			k. Ureter		
f. Renal artery					

PRONUNCIATIONS

Aorta (ay-OR-tah)
Aortic (ay-OR-tik)
Arterioles (ar-TEER-ee-ols)
Atria (AY-tri-uh)
Atrioventricular (AY-tree-oh-ven-TRIK-yoo-lar)
Autorhythmic (aw-toe-RITH-mik)
Calyces (KAY-lih-sees)
Capillaries (KAP-ih-layr-eez)
Coronary (KOR-oh-nayr-ee)
Diabetes insipidus (DIE-ah-BEET-ees in-SIP-ih-dus)
Dialysis (die-AL-ih-sis)
Diuretics (DIE-er-ET-iks)
Glomerulosclerosis (glom-AIR-yoo-lo-skler-OH-sis)
Glomerulus (gloh-MAYR-yoo-lus)
Henle (HEN-lee)
Hypokalemia (hie-poh-kay-LEE-mee-ah)
Hyponatremia (hie-poh-nay-TREE-mee-ah)
Lithotripsy (LITH-oh-TRIP-see)
Mitral (MY-trahl)
Nephropathy (nef-RAH-path-ee)
Pericardium (per-i-CAR-dee-um)
Purkinje (per-KIN-jee)
Retroperitoneal (RET-roh-payr-ih-ton-EE-al)
Sinoatrial (SI-noe-AY-tree-al)
Vasculature (VAS-cyoo-la-tur)
Vena cava (VEE-na KAY-va)
Ventricles (VEN-trik-uls)

Matching II

Match each electrolyte to its abbreviation. For additional study, write the range of normal serum values next to each.

Electrolytes	Abbreviation	Normal Serum Values
1. Bicarbonate		
2. Calcium		
3. Chloride		
4. Magnesium		
5. Phosphate		
6. Potassium		
7. Sodium		

ABBREVIATIONS

a. Ca^{2+}
b. Cl^-
c. HCO_3^-
d. K^+
e. Mg^{2+}
f. Na^+
g. PO_4^{-3}

Matching III

*Match each brand to its generic name and indication (either **D**=diuretic or **P**=potassium supplement). For additional study, write the type of diuretic or dosage form of potassium supplement beside each.*

Brand Names	Generic Names	Indi-cation	Type/Dosage Form
1. Aldactazide			
2. Aldactone			
3. Demadex			
4. Diamox			
5. Dyazide			
6. Kaon			
7. K-dur			
8. Klor-Con M			
9. Klorvess			
10. K-Tab			
11. Lasix			
12. Maxzide			
13. Midamor			
14. Moduretic			
15. Zaroxolyn			

GENERIC NAMES

a. acetazolamide
b. amiloride
c. amiloride/HCTZ
d. furosemide
e. metolazone
f. potassium bicarbonate
g. potassium chloride
h. potassium gluconate
i. spironolactone
j. spironolactone/HCTZ
k. torsemide
l. triamterene/HCTZ

True or False

For additional study, try to change the false statements to make them true.

_____1. The human heart has four chambers; two are ventricles and two are vena cava.

_____2. When the heart's electrical system malfunctions, abnormal heartbeats, termed arrhythmia, may occur.

_____3. The capillaries are the smallest of the blood vessels and connect the arterial and venous systems.

_____4. Arteries have valves that prevent blood from flowing backward or pooling in the extremities.

_____5. The rate at which the water and solutes from the blood are filtered into the renal tubule is termed tubular secretion.

_____6. Potassium is the most abundant cation in the body.

_____7. Anions carry a positive charge and include chlorine and phosphate.

_____8. Diuretics are often important in the treatment of hypertension.

_____9. Desmopressin is a synthetic form of the natural antidiuretic hormone.

_____10. Hypertensive nephropathy refers to the kidney damage caused by medications such as NSAIDs.

Short Answer

1. What is coronary artery disease, and why can it be life-threatening?

2. What is the importance of electrolyte homeostasis, and how is the kidney involved in this process?

3. Why are potassium products often prescribed for patients who are taking diuretics?

4. What is a normal body pH, and what does it mean? Which electrolyte is important in maintaining pH?

5. What is a kidney stone? How does it form, and what problems can it cause?

DRUG MONOGRAPH

*Choose one brand-name diuretic from **Medication Table 13-2** and complete a drug monograph using the form provided here. (An example of the drug monograph is included in Chapter 1 of this workbook.)*

Generic Name _____

Brand Name _____

Manufacturer _____

APPROVED INDICATION(S)

_____

_____

_____

_____

DOSAGE AND ROUTE(S) OF ADMINISTRATION

_____

_____

_____

AVAILABLE DOSAGE FORM(S) STRENGTH(S)

STORAGE/HANDLING CONDITIONS/PROCEDURES

_____

_____

_____

PRECAUTIONS (CONTRAINDICATIONS, DRUG/FOOD INTERACTIONS, PREGNANCY CATEGORY)

_____

_____

_____

_____

_____

_____

COMMON OR SEVERE ADVERSE REACTIONS

_____

_____

_____

_____

_____

INSTRUCTIONS FOR PATIENTS

_____

_____

_____

_____

COST OF THERAPY (DAILY, MONTHLY, FULL COURSE)

_____

_____

_____

OTHER DRUGS IN THIS CLASS

_____

_____

ADDITIONAL MEDICATIONS WITH SAME INDICATION

_____

_____

_____

ADVANTAGES/DISADVANTAGES COMPARED TO DRUGS LISTED ABOVE (CLASS, INDICATION)

_____

_____

_____

_____

_____

CHAPTER 14

Hypertension

LEARNING OBJECTIVES

After completing this chapter, you should be able to

1. Define the terms blood pressure and hypertension

2. Describe the various mechanisms used by the body to regulate blood pressure

3. List the blood pressure values associated with each blood pressure classification

4. Identify the consequences of untreated hypertension

5. Explain nonpharmacological strategies used to treat hypertension

6. Describe the mechanism of action, typical dosing, and side effects of the commonly used antihypertensive agents

7. State the brand and generic names and pharmacological classes of the most commonly used antihypertensive agents and combinations

Matching I

Match each brand name beta blocker with its generic name. For additional study, identify each as **S** *(cardioselective),* **N** *(non-selective),* **ISA** *(intrinsic sympathomimetic activity), or* **M** *(mixed alpha and beta blocker).*

Brand Names	Generic Names	S, N, ISA, or M
1. Brevibloc		
2. Bystolic		
3. Coreg		
4. Corgard		
5. Inderal		
6. InnoPran XL		
7. Lopressor		
8. Sectral		
9. Tenormin		
10. Toprol XL		
11. Trandate		
12. Zebeta		

GENERIC NAMES

a. acebutolol
b. atenolol
c. bisoprolol
d. carvedilol
e. esmolol
f. labetalol
g. metoprolol
h. nadolol
i. nebivolol
j. propranolol

PRONUNCIATIONS

Aldosterone (al-DOS-ter-ohn)

Angiotensin I (an-jee-oh-TEN-sin one)

Angiotensinogen (an-jee-oh-ten-SIN-oh-jen)

Diastole (die-ASS-toh-lee)

Diastolic (DIE-ah-STAH-lik)

Dihydropyridines (die-hie-droh-peer-ih-deenz)

Edema (eh-DEE-mah)

Hypertrophied (hi-PER-troh-feed)

Hyperuricemia (hie-per-yoor-ih-SEE-mee-ah)

Renin (REE-nin)

Retinopathy (ret-in-OP-ah-thee)

Sphygmomanometer (sfig-moh-man-OM-eh-ter)

Systole (SIS-toh-lee)

Systolic (sis-TAH-lik)

Matching II

*Match each brand name antihypertensive with its generic name and its type (**ACEI** or **ARB**).*

Brand Names	Generic Names	Type (ACEI or ARB)
1. Accupril		
2. Aceon		
3. Altace		
4. Atacand		
5. Avapro		
6. Benicar		
7. Cozaar		
8. Diovan		
9. Lotensin		
10. Mavik		
11. Micardis		
12. Prinivil		
13. Univasc		
14. Vasotec		
15. Zestril		

GENERIC NAMES

a. benazepril

b. candesartan

c. enalapril

d. irbesartan

e. lisinopril

f. losartan

g. moexipril

h. olmesartan

i. perindopril

j. quinapril

k. ramipril

l. telmisartan

m. trandolapril

n. valsartan

Matching III

Match each brand name antihypertensive with its generic name and class. For additional study, note whether the preparations are extended release or if they are available as injections.

Brand Names	Generic Names	Class	Extended Release/ Injection
1. Adalat CC			
2. Calan SR			
3. Cardene			
4. Cardura XL			
5. Cartia XT			
6. Catapres			
7. Cleviprex			
8. Covera HS			
9. Dilacor XR			
10. Nitropress			
11. Norvasc			
12. Procardia XL			
13. Tenex			
14. Tiazac			
15. Verelan PM			

GENERIC NAMES

a. amlodipine

b. clevidipine

c. clonidine

d. diltiazem

e. doxazosin

f. guanfacine

g. nicardipine

h. nifedipine

i. nitroprusside

j. verapamil

CLASS

K: Alpha antagonist

L: Central alpha agonist

V: Vasodilator

CCB: Calcium channel blocker

Matching IV

Match each side effect with the antihypertensives that may cause it.

Side Effects	Drug Class(es)
1. Angioedema	
2. Asthma	
3. Bradycardia	
4. Congestive heart failure	
5. Dizziness	
6. Dry cough	
7. Edema	
8. Headache	
9. Hyperglycemia	
10. Hyperkalemia	
11. Hyperuricemia	
12. Impotence	
13. Kidney failure	
14. Orthostatic hypotension	
15. Reflex tachycardia	

DRUG CLASS

a. Angiotensin II converting enzyme inhibitors (ACEIs)
b. Angiotensin II receptor blockers (ARBs)
c. Cardioselective beta adrenergic blockers
d. Nonselective beta blockers
e. Dihydropyridine calcium channel blockers
f. Non-dihydropyridine calcium channel blockers
g. Thiazide diuretics

True or False

For additional study, try to change the false statements to make them true.

_____1. Blood pressure is regulated by an interaction of many body organs and systems, including the heart and the kidneys.

_____2. High blood pressure resulting from conditions such as kidney disease or hyperthyroidism is known as primary hypertension.

_____3. A patient with a systolic blood pressure of 125 and a diastolic reading of 81 ("125/81") would be said to have prehypertension.

_____4. Medications are the only effective treatment for hypertension.

_____5. Thiazides are reserved for the treatment of hypertensive patients who are unable to afford more effective therapy.

_____6. Cardioselective beta blockers have more side effects on more body systems than nonselective blockers.

_____7. Patients taking some calcium channel blockers are warned to limit their intake of grapefruit juice because it interferes with the liver's ability to metabolize these agents.

_____8. Clonidine is an antihypertensive agent that can be administered either orally or as a transdermal patch.

_____9. Hypertrichosis, or excess hair growth, is a side effect of the antihypertensive hydralazine.

_____10. When pregnant patients must be treated for hypertension, ACE inhibitors are the usual choice.

Short Answer

1. Why should hypertension be treated even if patients feel healthy and do not have symptoms?

2. What is the reason combination products are prescribed for patients with hypertension? What are the disadvantages of this type of therapy?

3. Name the generic medications combined with hydro-chlorothiazide (HCTZ) in the following antihypertensive products: Avalide, Hyzaar, Prinzide, Zestoretic. To what class of medication does each belong?

4. What are some of the factors that figure into a physician's decisions regarding which types of antihypertensive agents to prescribe for a particular patient?

5. What are the types of hypertensive crises patients may suffer if their condition is not controlled? How is it treated?

DRUG MONOGRAPH

*Choose one brand-name anithypertensive combination from **Medication Table 14-5** and complete a drug monograph using the form provided here. (An example of the drug monograph is included in Chapter 1 of this workbook.)*

Generic Name _____

Brand Name _____

Manufacturer _____

APPROVED INDICATION(S)

_____

_____

_____

_____

DOSAGE AND ROUTE(S) OF ADMINISTRATION

_____

_____

_____

AVAILABLE DOSAGE FORM(S) STRENGTH(S)

STORAGE/HANDLING CONDITIONS/PROCEDURES

_____

_____

_____

PRECAUTIONS (CONTRAINDICATIONS, DRUG/FOOD INTERACTIONS, PREGNANCY CATEGORY)

_____

_____

_____

_____

_____

COMMON OR SEVERE ADVERSE REACTIONS

_____

_____

_____

_____

_____

INSTRUCTIONS FOR PATIENTS

_____

_____

_____

_____

COST OF THERAPY (DAILY, MONTHLY, FULL COURSE)

_____

_____

_____

OTHER DRUGS IN THIS CLASS

_____

_____

_____

ADDITIONAL MEDICATIONS WITH SAME INDICATION

_____

_____

_____

ADVANTAGES/DISADVANTAGES COMPARED TO DRUGS LISTED ABOVE (CLASS, INDICATION)

_____

_____

_____

_____

CHAPTER 15

Heart Disease

LEARNING OBJECTIVES

After completing this chapter, you should be able to

1. Define ischemic heart disease, acute coronary syndrome, heart failure, arrhythmia, and shock and identify their causes, symptoms, and consequences

2. List the nonpharmacologic treatments for the heart diseases above

3. Identify the various pharmacological treatments used to treat heart diseases and their basic mechanisms of action

4. Describe the common side effects caused by each of the medication classes used to treat heart diseases

Matching I

Match each definition to its term. For additional study, if the term has a common abbreviation, write it in the margin.

Definitions	Terms	Abbrev.
1. Abnormal pattern of heart beats		
2. Blocked coronary arteries resulting in insufficient oxygen to heart		
3. Blocked coronary arteries resulting in myocardial cell death		
4. Bypass of blocked coronary arteries using blood vessels from patient's legs		
5. Cardiac output insufficient for the body's needs		
6. Graphic representation of heart's electrical activity		
7. Insufficient blood flow resulting from damage to heart		
8. Life-threatening cardiovascular emergency		
9. Placement of a stent to open blocked coronary arteries		
10. Procedure to visualize and/or open blocked coronary arteries		
11. Relating to cardiac contractility		
12. Slower than normal heart rate		

TERMS

a. Acute coronary syndrome
b. Arrhythmia
c. Bradycardia
d. Cardiac catheterization
e. Cardiogenic shock
f. Coronary artery bypass graft
g. Electrocardiogram
h. Heart failure
i. Inotropic
j. Ischemic heart disease
k. Myocardial infarction
l. Percutaneous coronary intervention

PRONUNCIATIONS

Angina (ANN-jin-ah)
Arrhythmias (aye-RITH-mee-ahs)
Diaphoresis (die-ah-for-EE-sis)
Electrocardiogram (ee-lek-troh-KAR-dee-oh-gram)
Fibrinolytic (fie-brin-oh-LIT-ik)
Ischemic (iss-KEY-mik)
Myocardial infarctions (MY-oh-KAR-dee-all in-FARK-shuns)
Syncope (SIN-ko-pee)
Troponin (troe-POE-nin)
Vasospasms (VAY-zo-spaz-ums)

Matching II

Match each brand name medication used for ACS to its generic name and the class to which it belongs

Brand Names	Generic Names	Class
1. Activase		
2. Aggrastat		
3. Ecotrin		
4. Fragmin		
5. Integrilin		
6. Lovenox		
7. Plavix		
8. ReoPro		
9. Retavase		
10. TNKase		

GENERIC NAMES

a. abciximab   f. enoxaparin

b. alteplase   g. eptifibatide

c. aspirin   h. reteplase

d. clopidogrel   i. tenecteplase

e. dalteparin   j. tirofiban

CLASS

AP =   Antiplatelet agent

CB =   Fibrinolytic ("Clot buster")

GI =   Glycoprotein IIB/IIIA inhibitor

LMWH = Low molecular weight heparin

Matching III

Match each brand name nitrate to its generic and dosage form. For additional study, note which are long acting (once or twice daily) by placing the letters LA next to them.

Brand Names	Generic Names	Dosage	Long Acting
1. Dilatrate-SR			
2. Imdur			
3. Isordil			
4. Minitran			
5. Nitro-Bid			
6. Nitro-Dur			
7. Nitrolingual			
8. Nitrostat			
9. Nitro-Time			

GENERIC NAMES

a. isosorbide dinitrate

b. isosorbide mononitrate

c. nitroglycerin

DOSAGE FORMS

PC =   PO capsule   **TO =**   transdermal ointment

PT =   PO tablet   **TP =**   transdermal patch

SL =   sublingual tab   **TL =**   translingual spray

Matching IV

Match each brand name antiarrhythmic to its generic name and route(s) of administration. For additional study, write the Type (IA, etc.) of each antiarrthymic drug in the extra space.

Brand Names	Generic Names	Route(s) of Administration	Type
1. Betapace			
2. Calan			
3. Cordarone			
4. Corvert			
5. Multaq			
6. Norpace			
7. Rythmol			
8. Tambocor			
9. Tikosyn			
10. Xylocaine			

GENERIC NAMES

a. amiodarone

b. disopyramide

c. dofetilide

d. dronedarone

e. flecainide

f. ibutilide

g. lidocaine

h. propafenone

i. sotalol

j. verapamil

True or False

For additional study, try to change the false statements to make them true.

_____1. Ischemic heart disease is always accompanied by chest pain symptoms (angina).

_____2. In addition to nitrates, medications for treatment of angina include many of the same drugs used to treat hypertension, including beta blockers and calcium channel blockers.

_____3. Erectile dysfunction medications, such as Viagra, should not be taken by patients who are also on nitrate therapy.

_____4. If PCI or CABG is not available, the first goal of treatment for patients suffering from STEMI acute coronary syndrome is to relieve their pain, often with a combination of nitroglycerin and morphine.

_____5. Among antiarrhythmics, procainamide is notorious for causing severe gastrointestinal complaints including vomiting, diarrhea, and abdominal cramping, and quinidine has been implicated as a cause of systemic lupus erythematosus.

_____6. Lidocaine is so effective in controlling ventricular arrhythmias that it is routinely used in both the hospital and outpatient settings.

_____7. Because clopidogrel increases the risk of bleeding, patients who have been treated with this agent cannot undergo CABG until at least 5 days after the medication has been discontinued.

_____8. African Americans are among the patients for whom the combination of hydralazine and isosorbide dinitrate can be an effective heart failure treatment.

_____9. Fluids used in the treatment of shock, including albumin, hetastarch, and dextran, are sometimes known as crystalloids.

_____10. ACLS stands for advanced cardiac life support and involves advanced assessment and monitoring techniques (such as the EKG), placement of airway and intravenous access devices, and administration of medications.

Short Answer

1. What cautions and procedures specific to sublingual nitroglycerin tablets must technicians keep in mind when dispensing them?

2. Why do many emergency departments stock a fibrinolytic for ready use on admission of a patient with suspected stroke or acute coronary syndrome instead of waiting for the pharmacy department to supply it?

3. How does digoxin work, and what are its advantages in the treatment of heart failure? Why is it no longer the drug of choice?

4. What is a positive inotrope? Name two examples and their mechanisms of action.

5. What medications are most likely to be used in emergencies and, thus, kept in a crash cart?

DRUG MONOGRAPH

*Choose one brand-name nitrate product from **Medication Table 15-1** and complete a drug monograph using the form provided here. (An example of the drug monograph is included in Chapter 1 of this workbook.)*

Generic Name _____

Brand Name _____

Manufacturer _____

APPROVED INDICATION(S)

_____
_____
_____
_____

DOSAGE AND ROUTE(S) OF ADMINISTRATION

_____
_____
_____

AVAILABLE DOSAGE FORM(S) STRENGTH(S)

STORAGE/HANDLING CONDITIONS/PROCEDURES

_____
_____
_____

PRECAUTIONS (CONTRAINDICATIONS, DRUG/FOOD INTERACTIONS, PREGNANCY CATEGORY)

_____
_____
_____
_____

COMMON OR SEVERE ADVERSE REACTIONS

_____
_____
_____
_____
_____

INSTRUCTIONS FOR PATIENTS

_____
_____
_____
_____

COST OF THERAPY (DAILY, MONTHLY, FULL COURSE)

_____
_____

OTHER DRUGS IN THIS CLASS

_____
_____
_____

ADDITIONAL MEDICATIONS WITH SAME INDICATION

_____
_____
_____

ADVANTAGES/DISADVANTAGES COMPARED TO DRUGS LISTED ABOVE (CLASS, INDICATION)

_____
_____
_____
_____
_____

CHAPTER 16

Hyperlipidemia

LEARNING OBJECTIVES

After completing this chapter, you should be able to

1. Define hyperlipidemia and recognize its causes, symptoms, and consequences
2. Identify tests for hyperlipidemias and recognize the conditions under which they are done
3. Distinguish between total cholesterol, LDL, HDL, VLDL, and triglycerides, know the meaning of each acronym, and recognize target values for each
4. List nonpharmacologic treatments recommended for each type of hyperlipidemia
5. List the classes of medications used in the treatment of hyperlipidemia and their basic mechanisms of action
6. Identify agents and common side effects from each class of medications used to treat hyperlipidemias

PRONUNCIATIONS

Bile acid sequestrants (bie-ul ASS-id see-KWES-trantz)

Cholesterol (koe-LESS-ter-ol)

Chylomicrons (kie-loh-MIE-kronz)

Hyperlipidemia (hi-per-lip-id-EE-mee-ah)

Lipoproteins (lie-poh-PRO-teen)

Triglycerides (try-GLIH-ser-eyed)

Matching I

Match each side/adverse effect to its medication class.

Side/Adverse Effects	Medication Class(es)
1. Bloating, belching	
2. Blood glucose elevation	
3. Constipation, flatulence	
4. Fishy aftertaste	
5. Flushing	
6. Liver damage	
7. Myalgia (muscle pain)	
8. Nausea, vomiting, diarrhea, heartburn	
9. Rhabdomyolysis	
10. Upset stomach	

MEDICATION CLASSES

a. Bile acid sequestrant

b. Fibrates

c. Niacins

d. Omega 3

e. Statins

Matching II

Match each brand name hyperlipidemia medication to its generic name and class. For additional study, write the available dosage form(s) for each agent.

Brand Names	Generic Names	Class	Dosage Form(s)
1. Antara			
2. Colestid			
3. Crestor			
4. Lescol			
5. Lipitor			
6. Lipofen			
7. Livalo			
8. Lofibra			
9. Lopid			
10. Lovaza			
11. Mevacor			
12. Pravachol			
13. Prevalite			
14. Questran			
15. Tricor			
16. Triglide			
17. Trilipix			
18. Welchol			
19. Zetia			
20. Zocor			

GENERIC NAMES

a. atorvastatin   f. fenofibrate   k. pitavastatin

b. cholestyramine   g. fish oil   l. pravastatin

c. colesevelam   h. fluvastatin   m. rosuvastatin

d. colestipol   i. gemfibrozil   n. simvastatin

e. ezetimibe   j. lovastatin

CLASSES

Bile acid sequestrant

Cholesterol absorption inhibitor

Fibrate

Omega-3 fatty acid

Statin

True or False

For additional study, try to change the false statements to make them true.

_____1. All lipids in the human body can be classified as cholesterol.

_____2. Cholesterol is an important component of cell membranes.

_____3. LDL (low density lipoprotein) is known as good cholesterol because elevated levels are associated with a lower risk of developing heart disease.

_____4. Cholesterol and triglyceride concentrations in the blood reflect only those that are consumed in the diet.

_____5. Bile acid sequestrants are the preferred agents for treating hyperlipidemia in pregnant women.

_____6. Statins work by blocking an enzyme used by the body in its production of cholesterol.

_____7. Patients may not gain the full effect of the fibrates until they have completed 6–8 weeks of therapy.

_____8. Fenofibrate comes in several brand-name formulations that can be interchanged as generic equivalents.

_____9. Ezetimibe is classified as a HMG-CoA inhibitor (statin).

_____10. Omega 3 fatty acids can lower LDL cholesterol by as much as 50%.

Short Answer

1. Describe the Therapeutic Lifestyle Changes (TLC) Diet recommended to reduce LDL cholesterol.

2. What are the pleiotropic effects of the HMG-CoA inhibitors used for hyperlipidemia?

3. What are the differences between immediate-release and sustained-release niacin products?

4. What factors and characteristics limit the use of ezetimibe in the treatment of hyperlipidemia?

5. What instructions should be given to patients who are taking additional medications as well as a bile acid sequestrant such as Questran (cholestyramine)? Why?

DRUG MONOGRAPH

Choose one brand-name HMG-CoA reducatase inhibitor (statin) from Medication Table 16-1 and complete a drug monograph using the form provided here. (An example of the drug monograph is included in Chapter 1 of this workbook.)

Generic Name _____

Brand Name _____

Manufacturer _____

APPROVED INDICATION(S)

_____

_____

_____

_____

DOSAGE AND ROUTE(S) OF ADMINISTRATION

_____

_____

_____

AVAILABLE DOSAGE FORM(S) STRENGTH(S)

STORAGE/HANDLING CONDITIONS/PROCEDURES

_____

_____

PRECAUTIONS (CONTRAINDICATIONS, DRUG/FOOD INTERACTIONS, PREGNANCY CATEGORY)

_____

_____

_____

_____

_____

COMMON OR SEVERE ADVERSE REACTIONS

_____

_____

_____

_____

_____

INSTRUCTIONS FOR PATIENTS

_____

_____

_____

_____

COST OF THERAPY (DAILY, MONTHLY, FULL COURSE)

_____

_____

_____

OTHER DRUGS IN THIS CLASS

_____

_____

_____

ADDITIONAL MEDICATIONS WITH SAME INDICATION

_____

_____

_____

_____

ADVANTAGES/DISADVANTAGES COMPARED TO DRUGS LISTED ABOVE (CLASS, INDICATION)

_____

_____

_____

_____

CHAPTER 17

Overview of the Respiratory System

LEARNING OBJECTIVES

After completing this chapter, you should be able to

1. Identify components of the upper and lower respiratory systems
2. Recall basic physiology of respiratory system
3. Describe the process of respiratory gas exchange between oxygen and carbon dioxide and explain its importance
4. Identify and explain the different respiratory function tests that are used to evaluate respiratory function
5. Describe proper technique for administration of medication via respiratory routes

Matching I

Match each label to the part of the respiratory system it represents. For additional study, write the function of the structure next to the label.

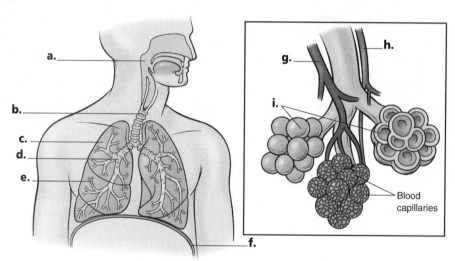

Blood capillaries

Part	Letter	Function
1. Alveoli		
2. Bronchiole		
3. Bronchus		
4. Diaphragm		
5. Lung		
6. Pharynx		
7. Pulmonary artery		
8. Pulmonary vein		
9. Trachea		

PRONUNCIATIONS

Alveolar (al-VEE-oh-ler)
Alveoli (al-VEE-o-lye)
Bronchi (BRONG-ki)
Bronchial (brong-ke-el)
Bronchioles (BRONG-kee-olz)
Bronchus (BRONG-kus)
Carina (KUH-ree-nuh)
Cilia (SILL-ee-uh)
Epiglottis (eh-pi-GLOT-iss)
Epithelial (ep-i-THEE-lee-al)
Hemoglobin (HEE-mo-gloe-bin)
Inspiratory (in-SPY-ruh-tor-ee)
Laryngopharynx (lar-ING-o-fair-inks)
Larynx (LAYR-inks)
Mediastinum (me-dee-uh-STY-nem)
Nasopharynx (NAY-zoe-fair-inks)
Nebulizer (NEB-yoo-lize-er)
Nebulizers (NEB-yoo-lize-ers)
Oropharynx (OR-o-fair-inks)
Pharynx (FAIR-inks)
Pleura (PLOOR-a)
Pleural (PLOOR-ul)
Spirometry (spi-ROM-i-tree)
Thoracic diaphragm (thor-ASS-ik DIE-uh-fram)
Trachea (TRAY-kee-uh)

Matching II

Match each definition to its term. For additional study, indicate any common abbreviations used for the terms.

Definitions	Terms	Abbreviation
1. Amount of air exhaled with force after maximum inhalation		
2. Device that delivers aerosolized medication to the lungs		
3. Device to deliver medications to the lungs as a fine mist using a compressor		
4. Device used to deliver medication to the lungs without an aerosol propellant		
5. Measure of oxygen and carbon dioxide in the blood		
6. Tests of lung function		
7. Tube which connects to the mouthpiece of an inhaler to increase the amount of medication reaching the lungs		

TERMS

a. Arterial blood gas
b. Dry powder inhaler
c. Forced vital capacity
d. Metered dose inhaler
e. Nebulizer
f. Pulmonary function tests
g. Spacer

True or False

For additional study, try to change the false statements to make them true.

_____1. Breathing accomplishes the inhalation of oxygen and the exhalation of carbon dioxide.

_____2. Oxygen is a waste product of cellular metabolism.

_____3. The pharynx functions as part of both the respiratory and the digestive systems.

_____4. Nebulizers are not suitable for use by children or the elderly.

_____5. Dry powder inhalers may be stored indefinitely as long as they are kept away from heat after the pouch is opened.

_____6. Forced expiratory volume (FEV) refers to the maximum amount of air exhaled forcefully in one breath.

_____7. Spacers are often recommended to decrease the amount of drug the patient will take into the lungs.

_____8. Dry powder inhalers should be primed before the first use by expelling one dose.

_____9. Improper inhaler technique can result in delivery to the gastrointestinal tract of medications intended for the lungs.

_____10. Dry powder inhalers usually require electricity from an outlet or battery to deliver medication.

Short Answer

1. Why is inhalation the preferred route of administration for the treatment of many respiratory conditions?

2. What should patients do after each inhalation of a corticosteroid, and why?

3. Describe cleaning instructions for metered dose inhalers used with spacers.

CHAPTER 18

Disorders of the Respiratory System

LEARNING OBJECTIVES

After completing this chapter, you should be able to

1. Define asthma, chronic obstructive pulmonary disease, and cystic fibrosis
2. Recall the pathophysiology of asthma, chronic obstructive pulmonary disease, and cystic fibrosis
3. List nonpharmacologic therapy options for asthma, chronic obstructive pulmonary disease, and cystic fibrosis
4. List pharmacotherapy options for asthma, chronic obstructive pulmonary disease, and cystic fibrosis
5. Recognize differences in asthma and chronic obstructive pulmonary disease pharmacotherapy
6. State generic and brand names of medications used to treat asthma, chronic obstructive pulmonary disease, and cystic fibrosis
7. Recognize the doses and side effects of pharmacologic therapies for disorders of the respiratory system

PRONUNCIATIONS

Bronchoconstriction (BRON-koh-kun-STRIK-shun)

Exacerbation (ekz-ass-er-BAY-shun)

Matching I

Match each brand name medication to its generic name and route of administration. For additional study, mark each according to its indication(s) for asthma (**A**) or chronic obstructive pulmonary disease (**COPD**) and note the dosage form of any inhalations.

Brand Names	Generic Name	Route	Indica-tion(s)	Dosage Form
1. Accolate				
2. Aerobid				
3. Asmanex				
4. Atrovent				
5. Flovent				
6. ProAir HFA				
7. Pulmicort				
8. QVAR				
9. Serevent				
10. Singulair				
11. Spiriva				
12. Ventolin HFA				
13. Xolair				
14. Xopenex				
15. Zyflo				

GENERIC NAMES

a. albuterol
b. beclomethasone
c. budesonide
d. flunisolide
e. fluticasone
f. ipratropium
g. levalbuterol
h. mometasone
i. montelukast
j. omalizumab
k. salmeterol
l. tiotropium
m. zafirlukast
n. zileuton

ROUTES

O = Oral
P = Inhalation
Q = Injection

Fill-In

Complete the chart below by adding the generic names of the ingredients of these brand name bronchodilator combination products. Include the name of the beta agonist and the category of the medication that is **NOT** a bronchodilator.

Brand Names	Beta Agonist	Other Ingredient	Category
1. Advair			
2. Combivent			
3. Dulera			
4. Symbicort			

True or False

For additional study, try to change the false statements to make them true.

_____1. Patients with asthma and COPD should receive yearly immunizations against influenza and pneumonia.

_____2. Asthma symptoms such as coughing, wheezing, shortness of breath, and chest tightness are a result of the inflammation caused by a hypersensitivity reaction.

_____3. Chronic asthma is the term used for severe asthma symptoms that can progress quickly to an emergent, potentially fatal situation.

_____4. LABA medications should be used to treat asthma only as part of combination therapy and are never considered for use as rescue medications for acute asthma attacks.

_____5. Inhaled corticosteroids should be used only as part of combination therapy for the treatment of asthma and are never considered for use as rescue medications for acute asthma attacks.

_____6. Inhaled mast cell stabilizer medications such as cromolyn and nedocromil are never considered for use as rescue medications for acute asthma attacks.

_____7. Anticholinergic inhalers for treatment of COPD are available in both short- and long-acting formulations.

_____8. Inhaled corticosteroids should be used only as part of combination therapy for the treatment of COPD.

_____9. Cystic fibrosis is an inherited disease and affects many body organs, including the lungs and pancreas.

_____10. Cystic fibrosis patients often require lower doses of antibiotics because they typically have a slower clearance rate than patients without CF.

Short Answer

1. Describe the typical course of asthma.

2. In chronic asthma, what is the typical time between remission and exacerbation, and what factors might bring on exacerbation?

3. What is the role of quick-relief medications in the management of asthma? By what other term are they described?

4. What role do beta agonists play in the treatment of COPD? Which ones are preferred?

5. Why is pancreatic enzyme replacement necessary for CF patients? What symptoms are characteristic of pancreatic enzyme deficiency?

DRUG MONOGRAPH

*Choose one brand-name bronchodilator from **Medication Table 18-1** and complete a drug monograph using the form provided here. (An example of the drug monograph is included in Chapter 1 of this Workbook.)*

Generic Name _____

Brand Name _____

Manufacturer _____

APPROVED INDICATION(S)

_____
_____
_____
_____

DOSAGE AND ROUTE(S) OF ADMINISTRATION

_____
_____
_____

AVAILABLE DOSAGE FORM(S) STRENGTH(S)

STORAGE/HANDLING CONDITIONS/PROCEDURES

_____
_____
_____

PRECAUTIONS (CONTRAINDICATIONS, DRUG/FOOD INTERACTIONS, PREGNANCY CATEGORY)

_____
_____
_____
_____
_____

COMMON OR SEVERE ADVERSE REACTIONS

_____
_____
_____
_____
_____
_____

INSTRUCTIONS FOR PATIENTS

_____
_____
_____
_____
_____

COST OF THERAPY (DAILY, MONTHLY, FULL COURSE)

_____
_____
_____

OTHER DRUGS IN THIS CLASS

_____
_____
_____

ADDITIONAL MEDICATIONS WITH SAME INDICATION

_____
_____
_____

ADVANTAGES/DISADVANTAGES COMPARED TO DRUGS LISTED ABOVE (CLASS, INDICATION)

_____
_____
_____
_____

CHAPTER 19

Acid-Related Diseases of the Upper Gastrointestinal Tract

LEARNING OBJECTIVES

After completing this chapter, you should be able to

1. Define the following:

   - Upper gastrointestinal tract
   - Dyspepsia
   - Gastritis
   - Gastric erosions
   - Peptic ulcer disease
   - Gastroesophageal reflux disease
   - Heartburn
   - Esophagitis
   - Hiatal hernia
   - Stress-related mucosal damage or stress ulcer

2. Describe the anatomy and normal physiology of the upper gastrointestinal tract and discuss the role of gastric acid in acid-related diseases

3. Identify the causes and risk factors for dyspepsia, peptic ulcer disease, gastroesophageal reflux disease, and upper gastrointestinal bleeding

4. List the most common signs, symptoms, and complications of dyspepsia, peptic ulcer disease, gastroesophageal reflux disease, and upper gastrointestinal bleeding

5. Describe the nonpharmacologic treatment of dyspepsia, peptic ulcer disease, and gastroesophageal reflux disease

6. Explain the pharmacotherapeutic effects of antacids, H_2-receptor antagonists, proton pump inhibitors, sucralfate, bismuth salts, and misoprostol, and list their most common side effects and drug interactions

7. State the brand and generic names of the most widely used antacids, H_2-receptor antagonists, proton pump inhibitors, sucralfate, bismuth salts, and misoprostol along with their routes of administration, available dosage forms, and common dosages

8. Recognize common drug regimens for the treatment of dyspepsia, peptic ulcer disease, gastroesophageal reflux disease, and upper gastrointestinal bleeding

PRONUNCIATIONS

Adenocarcinoma (ad-n-oh-kahr-suh-NOH-muh)

Ascites (uh-SIE-tes)

Dyspepsia (dis PEP see ah)

Endoscopy (en-DOS-kuh-pee)

Esophagus (ee-SOF-uh-guhs)

Gastroesophageal reflux (gas-troh-ee-SOF-uh-JEE-ul REE-fluks)

Gastroparesis (GAS-troh-puh-REE-sis)

Hypercalcemia (hie-per-cal-SEEM-ee-a)

Prostaglandins (pros-tuh-GLAN-dins)

Regurgitation (ri-gur-ji-TAY-shun)

Tachyphylaxis (TA-key-fil- AX-is)

Matching I

Match each brand product to its generic name and class (mechanism of action). For additional study, mark which drugs are available OTC.

Brand Names	Generic Names	Class	OTC?
1. Aciphex			
2. Axid AR			
3. Dexilant			
4. Nexium			
5. Pepcid AC			
6. Prevacid 24HR			
7. Prilosec			
8. Protonix			
9. Tagamet HB			
10. Zantac-150			

GENERIC NAMES

a. cimetidine	f. nizatidine
b. dexlansoprazole	g. omeprazole
c. esomeprazole	h. pantoprazole
d. famotidine	i. rabeprazole
e. lansoprazole	j. ranitidine

CLASS

PPI = Proton pump inhibitor

H2RA = Histamine-2 receptor antagonist

Matching II

Match each condition to its definition and indicate whether the pharmacist might recommend OTC products or a physician visit (referral) for treatment.

Conditions	Definition	OTC or Referral
1. Dyspepsia		
2. Gastroesopha-geal reflux disease		
3. Peptic ulcer disease		
4. Stress-related mucosal damage		

DEFINITIONS

a. Acute damage to the lining of the stomach of critically ill patients.

b. Damage to the stomach or duodenum extending into the submucosal layer and/or muscle tissues

c. Heartburn or esophageal injury caused by backward flow of stomach contents

d. Indigestion or abdominal discomfort with belching, bloating, and/or heartburn

True or False

For additional study, try to change the false statements to make them true.

_____1. Antacids work by inhibiting acid secretion in the stomach.

_____2. OTC antacids have the potential to interfere with the absorption of some prescription medications.

_____3. H_2 receptor antagonists work by inhibiting acid secretion in the stomach.

_____4. Proton pump inhibitors work by reacting with stomach acid to neutralize it.

_____5. Misoprostol is contraindicated for pregnant women because it can cause abortion.

_____6. Liquid bismuth preparations can cause blackening of the teeth.

_____7. Eradication of *H. pylori* and ulcer-healing requires treatment with at least two different drugs, including one to inhibit acid secretion and one antibiotic.

_____8. Non-gastrointestinal symptoms of GERD may include asthma or laryngitis.

_____9. Many patients with heartburn can get adequate treatment with OTC medications recommended by the pharmacist.

_____10. Stress-related mucosal bleeding is so rare among hospital patients that measures to prevent it are seldom considered cost effective.

Short Answer

1. Describe the anatomy (parts) of the upper gastrointestinal tract and the function of each part.

2. What distinguishes the two groups of medications used to treat acid-related UGI conditions? Name medications that belong in each group.

3. When is the best time for a patient to take a PPI dose? Why?

4. What common medications can cause peptic ulcers? How?

5. What are the symptoms of UGI bleeding, and why is it dangerous?

DRUG MONOGRAPH

*Choose one brand-name proton pump inhibitor from **Medication Table 19-1** and complete a drug monograph using the form provided here. (An example of the drug monograph is included in Chapter 1 of this workbook.)*

Generic Name _____

Brand Name _____

Manufacturer _____

APPROVED INDICATION(S)

_____

_____

_____

_____

DOSAGE AND ROUTE(S) OF ADMINISTRATION

_____

_____

_____

AVAILABLE DOSAGE FORM(S) STRENGTH(S)

STORAGE/HANDLING CONDITIONS/PROCEDURES

_____

_____

_____

PRECAUTIONS (CONTRAINDICATIONS, DRUG/FOOD INTERACTIONS, PREGNANCY CATEGORY)

_____

_____

_____

_____

_____

COMMON OR SEVERE ADVERSE REACTIONS

_____

_____

_____

_____

INSTRUCTIONS FOR PATIENTS

_____

_____

_____

_____

COST OF THERAPY (DAILY, MONTHLY, FULL COURSE)

_____

_____

OTHER DRUGS IN THIS CLASS

_____

_____

_____

ADDITIONAL MEDICATIONS WITH SAME INDICATION

_____

_____

_____

ADVANTAGES/DISADVANTAGES COMPARED TO DRUGS LISTED ABOVE (CLASS, INDICATION)

_____

_____

_____

_____

PART 7

CHAPTER 20

Nausea, Vomiting, and Upper GI Tract Motility Disorders

LEARNING OBJECTIVES

After completing this chapter, you should be able to

1. Define the following:

   - Antiemetic
   - Chemoreceptor trigger zone
   - Emesis
   - Gastroparesis
   - Motion sickness
   - Nausea
   - Vestibular
   - Vomiting

2. Identify the causes and risk factors for developing nausea/vomiting and gastroparesis

3. List the most common signs and symptoms of nausea/vomiting and gastroparesis

4. Describe nonpharmacologic therapies for nausea and vomiting

5. Explain the pharmacotherapeutic effects of antacids, histamine-2 receptor antagonists, anticholinergics, antihistamines, dopamine antagonists, cannabinoids, corticosteroids, benzodiazepines, serotonin antagonists, and neurokinin-1 receptor antagonists and list their most common side effects and major drug interactions

6. State the brand and generic names of the most widely used antiemetic and pro-motility medications, along with their routes of administration, dosage forms, and available doses

7. Recognize common regimens for the treatment of nausea, vomiting, and gastroparesis

PRONUNCIATIONS

Antiemetic (an-tee-eh-MET-ik)

Benzamides (BENZ-uh-miedz)

Butyrophenones (byoo-ter-oh-feh-NOHNZ)

Cannabinoids (kuh-NA-bi-noidz)

Chemoreceptor (kee-moh-ree-SEP-ter)

Dopaminergic (doh-puh-min-ER-jik)

Emesis (EM-uh-sis or eh-MEE-sis)

Histaminic (hiss-tuh-MIN-ik)

Neurokinin (nyor-oh-KIE-nin)

Phenothiazines (fee-noh-THIE-uh-zeenz)

Vestibular (ves-TIB-yoo-ler)

Matching

Match each brand name to its generic name and regulatory status (RX or OTC). For additional study, note the route(s) of administration.

Brand Names	Generic Names	Regulatory Status	Route(s) of Administration
1. Aloxi			
2. Antivert			
3. Anzemet			
4. Cesamet			
5. Compazine			
6. Dramamine			
7. Emend			
8. Emetrol			
9. Marinol			
10. Phenergan			
11. Reglan			
12. Tigan			
13. Transderm Scōp			
14. Zofran			

GENERIC NAMES

a. aprepitant
b. dimenhydrinate
c. dolasetron
d. dronabinol
e. meclizine
f. metoclopramide
g. nabilone
h. ondansetron
i. palonosetron
j. phosphorated carbohydrate solution
k. prochlorperazine
l. promethazine
m. scopolamine
n. trimethobenzamide

True or False

For additional study, try to change the false statements to make them true.

_____1. Vomiting is unpleasant but unlikely to have dangerous consequences.

_____2. Dietary approaches to nausea/vomiting, such as frequent small meals or high protein snacks, are frequently recommended for pregnant patients so they can avoid possible adverse medication effects on their unborn children.

_____3. A scopolamine patch can prevent motion sickness for up to 72 hours.

_____4. Cannabinoid antiemetics are controlled substances because they are chemically related to opiates like morphine and codeine.

_____5. Patients whose nausea and vomiting are accompanied by fever and diarrhea should always try OTC antiemetics before seeking treatment by a physician.

_____6. While chamomile and peppermint oil are considered natural remedies for nausea, they are considered dangerous and ineffective and should never be used.

_____7. Patients who regularly drink alcoholic beverages are less likely to experience nausea and vomiting from cancer chemotherapy.

_____8. Patients who are non-smokers are more likely to experience postoperative nausea and vomiting.

_____9. People who are vomiting because of motion sickness are best treated with an oral OTC product.

_____10. A diabetic patient suffering from gastroparesis (delayed gastric emptying) is usually treated with a prescription medication to speed the clearance of food from the esophagus and stomach.

Short Answer

1. Discuss the causes of nausea and vomiting.

2. What are the three types of nausea and vomiting associated with cancer chemotherapy? What are the characteristics of each?

3. What considerations are important in the choice of nausea/vomiting treatment during pregnancy? What are some of the agents that may be used?

4. What are some of the symptoms of gastroparesis, and what types of patients are most likely to suffer from it?

5. Which patients are most likely to benefit from OTC antiemetics recommended by the pharmacist?

DRUG MONOGRAPH

*Choose one brand-name antiemetic from **Medication Table 20-1** and complete a drug monograph using the form provided here. (An example of the drug monograph is included in Chapter 1 of this workbook.)*

Generic Name _____

Brand Name _____

Manufacturer _____

APPROVED INDICATION(S)

_____
_____
_____
_____

DOSAGE AND ROUTE(S) OF ADMINISTRATION

_____
_____
_____

AVAILABLE DOSAGE FORM(S) STRENGTH(S)

STORAGE/HANDLING CONDITIONS/PROCEDURES

_____
_____
_____

PRECAUTIONS (CONTRAINDICATIONS, DRUG/FOOD INTERACTIONS, PREGNANCY CATEGORY)

_____
_____
_____
_____
_____

COMMON OR SEVERE ADVERSE REACTIONS

_____
_____
_____
_____
_____
_____

INSTRUCTIONS FOR PATIENTS

_____
_____
_____
_____
_____

COST OF THERAPY (DAILY, MONTHLY, FULL COURSE)

_____
_____
_____

OTHER DRUGS IN THIS CLASS

_____
_____
_____

ADDITIONAL MEDICATIONS WITH SAME INDICATION

_____
_____
_____

ADVANTAGES/DISADVANTAGES COMPARED TO DRUGS LISTED ABOVE (CLASS, INDICATION)

_____
_____
_____
_____

CHAPTER 21

Lower Gastrointestinal Tract

LEARNING OBJECTIVES

After completing this chapter, you should be able to

1. Define the following:
   - Lower gastrointestinal tract
   - Duodenal ulcer
   - Appendicitis
   - Gastroenteritis
   - Colonoscopy
2. Review the anatomy and normal physiology of the lower gastrointestinal tract
3. Identify the causes, risk factors, and clinical presentation for diarrhea, constipation, hemorrhoids, inflammatory bowel disease, irritable bowel syndrome, flatulence, and parasitic infections
4. Review the treatment goals for diarrhea, constipation, hemorrhoids, inflammatory bowel disease, irritable bowel syndrome, flatulence, and parasitic infections
5. List the nonpharmacologic, pharmacologic, and alternative treatment for diarrhea, constipation, hemorrhoids, inflammatory bowel disease, irritable bowel syndrome, flatulence, and parasitic infections
6. Discuss the therapeutic effects, drug properties, dosages, and routes of administration for each class of medications listed above, and list their most common side effects and drug interactions

PRONUNCIATIONS

Anorectal (ay-noh-REK-tul)

Anthraquinone (an-thruh-kwuh-nohn)

Anti-inflammatory (AN ti-in-FLAM-muh-TOR-ee)

Antipruritics (an-tee-proo-RIT-ik)

Ascaris lumbricoides (lum-bri-COY-des)

Campylobacter (KAM-pi-loh-bak-ter)

Cecum (SEE-kum)

Clostridium difficile (klo-STRID-ee-um dif-uh-SEEL)

Colonoscopy (koh-luh-NOS-kuh-pee)

Defecation (def-ih-KAY-shun)

Duodenum (doo-OD-eh-num)

Fibromyalgia (FYE-broh-mye-AL-juh)

Gastroenteritis (GAS-troh-en-ter-IE-tis)

Hyperalgesia (hye-per-AL-jee-zhuh)

Ileocecal (ill-ee-oh-SEE-kal)

Ileum (ILL-ee-um)

Jejunum (jee-JOO-num)

Lactobacillus acidophilus (lak-toh-buh-SILL-us ass-ih-DOF-ill-us)

Megacolon (MEG-uh-coh-lun)

Melanosis coli (mel-uh-NOH-sis kO-ll)

Pancreatitis (pan-kree-uh-TAHY-tis)

Protozoa (proh-tuh-ZOH-uh)

Protozoal (proh-tuh-ZOH-ul)

Pyloric sphincter (pie-LOR-ik SFINGK-ter)

Ricinoleic (RYE-sin-oh-lay-ik)

Rotavirus (ROH-tuh-vahy-ruhs)

Salmonella (sal-muh-NEL-uh)

Sigmoidoscopy (sig-moi-DOS-kuh-pee)

Ulcerative colitis (UL-ser-uh-tiv koh-LYE-tis)

Vermiform appendix (VER-mih-form ah-PEN-diks)

Matching I

*Match each brand name to its generic name and indication (Constipation = **C**, Diarrhea = **D**). For additional study, note the regulatory status (**RX** or **OTC**).*

Brand Names	Generic Names	Indication	Regulatory Status
1. Benefiber			
2. Colace			
3. Dulcolax			
4. Enulose			
5. Ex-Lax			
6. Haley's M-O			
7. Imodium			
8. Konsyl			
9. Kristalose			
10. Lomotil			
11. Maltsupex			
12. Metamucil			
13. MiraLAX			
14. Pepto Bismol			
15. Senokot			

GENERIC NAMES

a. bisacodyl
b. bismuth subsalicylate
c. diphenoxylate/atropine
d. docusate
e. lactulose
f. loperamide
g. methylcellulose
h. polyethylene glycol
i. psyllium
j. senna
k. sorbitol/magnesium/
mineral oil

Matching II

Match each brand name to its generic name and indication.

Brand Names	Generic Names	Indication
1. Asacol		
2. Azulfidine		
3. Cimzia		
4. Colazal		
5. Dipentum		
6. Humira		
7. Lotronex		
8. Mylicon		
9. Pentasa		
10. Remicade		
11. Rowasa		
12. Tysabri		

GENERIC NAMES

a. adalimumab
b. alosetron
c. balsalazide
d. certolizumab
e. infliximab
f. mesalamine
g. natalizumab
h. olsalazine
i. simethicone
j. sulfasalazine

INDICATIONS

K = Flatulence
L = Inflammatory bowel disease
M = Irritable bowel syndrome

True or False

For additional study, try to change the false statements to make them true.

_____1. The most important treatment for acute diarrhea is beginning an antidiarrheal medication.

_____2. The pharmacist may recommend loperamide liquid as an OTC diarrhea treatment for a 6-month-old infant who cannot swallow the capsules.

_____3. Patients who are allergic to aspirin may also be allergic to bismuth subsalicylate.

_____4. Lomotil (diphenoxylate/atropine) is a controlled substance.

_____5. The pharmacist may recommend a probiotic preparation such as *Lactobacillus* as an OTC diarrhea treatment for a child.

_____6. Patients taking opioid medication for cancer pain often require antidiarrheal medications to maintain regular bowel function.

_____7. Stool softeners, such as docusate, stimulate defecation by drawing water into the bowel and promote local irritation, stimulating evacuation.

_____8. Hemorrhoids are frequently treated with stool softeners as well as with local agents applied to the painful area.

_____9. Irritable bowel syndrome is a form of inflammatory bowel disease.

_____10. Patients who are allergic to sulfonamides (sulfa) are likely to also be allergic to mesalamine.

Short Answer

1. What are probiotics? Why are they useful in the treatment of diarrhea?

2. What important information should patients taking psyllium and bulk-forming laxatives know and why?

3. Why are some medications that are used for rheumatoid arthritis also prescribed for Crohn's disease and ulcerative colitis?

4. Why is alosetron subject to a restricted prescribing program? Describe some of the features of this program that are of importance to pharmacy technicians involved in dispensing this drug.

5. How do currently available treatments for parasitic worm infections work?

DRUG MONOGRAPH

*Choose one brand-name medication from **Medication Table 21-1** for the treatment of inflammatory bowel disease and complete a drug monograph using the form provided here. (An example of the drug monograph is included in Chapter 1 of this workbook.)*

Generic Name _____

Brand Name _____

Manufacturer _____

APPROVED INDICATION(S)

_____

_____

_____

_____

DOSAGE AND ROUTE(S) OF ADMINISTRATION

_____

_____

_____

AVAILABLE DOSAGE FORM(S) STRENGTH(S)

STORAGE/HANDLING CONDITIONS/PROCEDURES

_____

_____

PRECAUTIONS (CONTRAINDICATIONS, DRUG/FOOD INTERACTIONS, PREGNANCY CATEGORY)

_____

_____

_____

_____

_____

COMMON OR SEVERE ADVERSE REACTIONS

_____

_____

_____

_____

_____

_____

INSTRUCTIONS FOR PATIENTS

_____

_____

_____

_____

COST OF THERAPY (DAILY, MONTHLY, FULL COURSE)

_____

_____

_____

OTHER DRUGS IN THIS CLASS

_____

_____

_____

ADDITIONAL MEDICATIONS WITH SAME INDICATION

_____

_____

_____

_____

ADVANTAGES/DISADVANTAGES COMPARED TO DRUGS LISTED ABOVE (CLASS, INDICATION)

_____

_____

_____

_____

CHAPTER 22

Hepatic and Pancreatic Disorders

LEARNING OBJECTIVES

After completing this chapter, you should be able to

1. Define the following:

   - Ascites
   - Cirrhosis
   - Encephalopathy
   - Esophageal varices
   - Hepatitis
   - Jaundice
   - Malabsorption
   - Pancreatitis
   - Portal hypertension
   - Pseudocyst

2. Recall common causes and complications of chronic liver disease
3. Review the role and mechanism of common drug treatments for cirrhosis
4. Review adverse effects and drug interactions for medications used in the treatment of chronic liver disease
5. Identify key patient counseling points for medications used to treat complications of chronic liver disease
6. Describe the anatomy and normal physiology of the liver and pancreas
7. Recognize common medications used in the management of acute pancreatitis
8. Review adverse effects, drug interactions, and key patient counseling points for medications used in the treatment of chronic pancreatitis

PRONUNCIATIONS

Amylase (AM-ill-ayss)

Ascites (uh-SIE-teez)

Bilirubin (bill-ee-ROO-bin)

Cholecystokinin (KOH-leh-SIS-tih-KYE-nin)

Edema (eh-DEE-mah)

Encephalopathy (en-sef-uh-LOP-uh-thee)

Fibrosis (fye-BROH-sis)

Gynecomastia (gie-nee-koh-MAS-tee-uh)

Hepatocyte (heh-PAT-oh-siet)

Jaundice (JON-dis)

Kupffer (KUP-fer)

Paracentesis (payr-uh-sen-TEE-sis)

Protease (PROH-tee-ayss)

Sinusoid (SIE-nyoo-soyd)

Steatorrhea (stee-at-or-EE-ya)

Varices (VAYR-ih-seez)

Matching I

Match each definition or description with the corresponding term.

DEFINITIONS

_____1. Abdominal organ responsible for synthesizing proteins, cholesterol, and bile

_____2. Abnormal accumulation of fluid in the abdominal cavity

_____3. Brain/nervous system dysfunction caused by ammonia and waste products in the blood

_____4. Enlarged veins in the upper GI tract, which may burst and bleed easily

_____5. Increased pressure in the main vein of the liver

_____6. Infection of ascitic fluid in the peritoneal cavity

_____7. Inflammation of the liver

_____8. Inflammation of the pancreas

_____9. Liver disease in which scar tissue replaces normal tissue

_____10. Organ that secretes insulin, glucagon, somatostatin, and some digestive enzymes

_____11. Substance that helps remove fat-soluble substances from the body and aids in intestinal fat absorption

_____12. Yellow discoloration of skin and eyes caused by bilirubin accumulation

TERMS

a. Ascites

b. Bile

c. Cirrhosis

d. Hepatic encephalopathy

e. Hepatitis

f. Jaundice

g. Liver

h. Pancreas

i. Pancreatitis

j. Portal hypertension

k. Spontaneous bacterial peritonitis

l. Varices

Matching II

*Match each brand name drug to its generic and note whether it is used to treat conditions associated with liver disease (**L**) or pancreatic disease (**P**). For additional study, identify the condition (e.g., ascites) each medication is used to treat.*

Brand Names	Generic Names	Disease Type	Condition
1. Aldactone			
2. Creon			
3. Enulose			
4. Inderal LA			
5. Lasix			
6. Neo-Fradin			
7. Noroxin			
8. Sandostatin			
9. Xifaxan			
10. Zenpep			

GENERIC NAMES

a. furosemide
b. lactulose
c. neomycin
d. norfloxacin
e. octreotide
f. pancrelipase
g. propranolol
h. rifaximin
i. spironolactone

True or False

For additional study, try to change the false statements to make them true.

_____1. Cirrhosis is also known as end stage liver disease.

_____2. Variceal bleeding is the term used to refer to increased pressure in the portal vein that results from cirrhosis.

_____3. The most common diuretic regimen for treating ascites is a combination of furosemide with a thiazide, usually hydrochlorothiazide (HCTZ).

_____4. The laxative agent lactulose is often used to treat hepatic encephalopathy, the change in mental function associated with liver disease.

_____5. Patients who develop spontaneous bacterial peritonitis as a complication of chronic liver disease should be treated with antibiotics on a continuous regimen for the rest of their lives.

_____6. Rifaximin is not as effective as lactulose, neomycin, and metronidazole for the treatment of SBP but is sometimes used because it is less expensive.

_____7. Octreotide is administered as an intravenous infusion for five days when used in the treatment of variceal bleeding.

_____8. Albumin infusions can help reduce blood volume and flow to the kidneys in patients with liver disease.

_____9. Pancreatic enzyme replacement must be accomplished by injection.

_____10. Vitamin supplements for patients with chronic pancreatitis usually have high concentrations of the fat soluble vitamins A, D, E, and K.

Short Answer

1. What are the major complications of cirrhosis?

2. How can lactulose be administered to hospitalized patients who are unable to swallow?

3. What antibiotics are typically administered to treat patients hospitalized with acute spontaneous bacterial peritonitis?

4. Why is albumin used sparingly in the treatment of complications of cirrhosis?

5. What adverse effect of pancreatic enzyme therapy may occur if doses are above the recommended level?

DRUG MONOGRAPH

*Choose one brand-name pancreatic enzyme replacement product from **Medication Table 22-1** and complete a drug monograph using the form provided here. (An example of the drug monograph is included in Chapter 1 of this workbook.)*

Generic Name _____

Brand Name _____

Manufacturer _____

APPROVED INDICATION(S)

_____

_____

_____

_____

DOSAGE AND ROUTE(S) OF ADMINISTRATION

_____

_____

_____

AVAILABLE DOSAGE FORM(S) STRENGTH(S)

STORAGE/HANDLING CONDITIONS/PROCEDURES

_____

_____

_____

PRECAUTIONS (CONTRAINDICATIONS, DRUG/FOOD INTERACTIONS, PREGNANCY CATEGORY)

_____

_____

_____

_____

_____

COMMON OR SEVERE ADVERSE REACTIONS

_____

_____

_____

_____

INSTRUCTIONS FOR PATIENTS

_____

_____

_____

_____

_____

COST OF THERAPY (DAILY, MONTHLY, FULL COURSE)

_____

_____

_____

OTHER DRUGS IN THIS CLASS

_____

_____

_____

ADDITIONAL MEDICATIONS WITH SAME INDICATION

_____

_____

_____

ADVANTAGES/DISADVANTAGES COMPARED TO DRUGS LISTED ABOVE (CLASS, INDICATION)

_____

_____

_____

_____

_____

CHAPTER 23

Nutritional Pharmacology

LEARNING OBJECTIVES

After completing this chapter, you should be able to

1. Identify the vitamins and minerals necessary to the human body, their functions, and key food sources
2. List the three energy nutrients and the calories they contribute to the dietary intake
3. List some reasons why nutritional and vitamin supplementation may be necessary
4. List benefits and risks of vitamin supplementation
5. Identify the components of nutrition support formulations
6. Review preparation and administration of nutrition support
7. Discuss obesity and list approved medication therapies for this condition

PRONUNCIATIONS

Amino (uh-MEE-noh)
Anorexiants (ann-or-REX-ee-untz)
Carbohydrates (kar-boh-HYE-drayts)
Cholesterol (ko-LESS-ter-ol)
Glycerol (GLISS-er-oll)
Lipase (LYE-payss)
Lipids (LIH-pidz)
Phospholipids (FOS-fo-LIH-pidz)
Triglyceride (trie-GLIS-er-ied)

Matching

Match each definition or description with the corresponding term.

DEFINITIONS

_____1. Building blocks of body tissues, composed of amino acid combinations

_____2. Class of nutrients that includes sugar, starch, and fiber

_____3. Class of substances that includes fats, phospholipids, and cholesterol

_____4. Essential nutrients needed in small amounts for body functions

_____5. Fats that are solid at room temperature

_____6. Form of fat with a glycerol base on which three fatty acids are attached

_____7. Inorganic elements used for body processes

_____8. Non-nutrient lipid made by (and present in) humans and animals, but not plants

TERMS

a. Carbohydrates
b. Cholesterol
c. Lipids
d. Minerals
e. Proteins
f. Saturated fats
g. Triglycerides
h. Vitamins

Fill-In

*Complete the table with the letter name and, if appropriate, number of each vitamin and note whether it is considered fat-soluble (**F**) or water-soluble (**W**). The first line has been completed as an example.*

Vitamins	Letter/Number	Type
Biotin	*B7*	*W*
Alpha tocopherol		
Ascorbic acid		
Beta carotene		
Calcitriol		
Cholecalciferol		
Cyanocobalamin		
Ergocalciferol		
Hydroxocobalamin		
Niacin		
Pantothenic acid		
Phytonadione		
Pyridoxine		
Retinol		
Riboflavin		
Thiamine		

True or False

For additional study, try to change the false statements to make them true.

_____1.   Of the energy nutrients, fats have the highest caloric density (most calories per gram).

_____2.   Patients should be advised to choose the vitamin supplement with the highest available level of fat-soluble vitamins.

_____3.   Because excess quantities of the B vitamins are eliminated in the urine, toxicity from them is rare.

_____4.   Vitamin supplements are natural dietary products so they need not be included on a patient's medication profile.

_____5.   Some vitamin and dietary supplements may have interactions with a patient's prescribed medication therapy.

_____6.   Enteral nutrition is a nutrient preparation administered intravenously.

_____7.   Total parenteral nutrition consists of a mixture of energy nutrients, vitamins, and minerals (electrolytes).

_____8.   The protein source for most parenteral nutrition is dextrose.

_____9.   Natural weight loss products, such as guarana extract and chromium picolinate, have recommended dosages endorsed by the FDA.

_____10. The FDA has approved several appetite suppressants for use in physician-supervised weight-loss regimens.

Short Answer

1.   List some types of people who might benefit from multiple vitamin and mineral supplementation.

2.   List two risks of vitamin supplementation.

3.   List four conditions in which nutrition support may be necessary.

4.   What is meant by "cycling" in the administration of parenteral nutrition? What are the advantages of this technique?

5.   What types of weight-loss therapies have been approved by the FDA? Give examples of each.

DRUG MONOGRAPH

*Choose one brand-name weight loss product from **Medication Table 23-2** and complete a drug monograph using the form provided here. (An example of the drug monograph is included in Chapter 1 of this workbook.)*

Generic Name _____

Brand Name _____

Manufacturer _____

APPROVED INDICATION(S)

_____

_____

_____

_____

DOSAGE AND ROUTE(S) OF ADMINISTRATION

_____

_____

_____

AVAILABLE DOSAGE FORM(S) STRENGTH(S)

STORAGE/HANDLING CONDITIONS/PROCEDURES

_____

_____

_____

PRECAUTIONS (CONTRAINDICATIONS, DRUG/FOOD INTERACTIONS, PREGNANCY CATEGORY)

_____

_____

_____

_____

_____

_____

COMMON OR SEVERE ADVERSE REACTIONS

_____

_____

_____

_____

_____

_____

INSTRUCTIONS FOR PATIENTS

_____

_____

_____

_____

_____

COST OF THERAPY (DAILY, MONTHLY, FULL COURSE)

_____

_____

_____

OTHER DRUGS IN THIS CLASS

_____

_____

_____

ADDITIONAL MEDICATIONS WITH SAME INDICATION

_____

_____

_____

ADVANTAGES/DISADVANTAGES COMPARED TO DRUGS LISTED ABOVE (CLASS, INDICATION)

_____

_____

_____

_____

_____

CHAPTER 24

Overview of the Hematologic System

LEARNING OBJECTIVES

After completing this chapter, you should be able to

1. Describe the developmental process of red blood cells, white blood cells, and platelets

2. List nutritional requirements for proper development of red blood cells

3. Explain the structure and function of red blood cells, white blood cells, and platelets

4. Describe the processes the body uses to achieve hemostasis: vasoconstriction, platelet plug formation, and the clotting cascade

5. List the utility of the most common laboratory tests of the blood

Matching I

Match each definition or description to the appropriate term.

DEFINITIONS

_____1. Blood cell protein that carries oxygen

_____2. Blood cell responsible for forming clots

_____3. Decreased number of white blood cells

_____4. Growth factor controlling production of red blood cells

_____5. Liquid component of blood

_____6. Mature red blood cell

_____7. Most common protein in plasma

_____8. Process of forming a blood clot

_____9. Storage form of iron in the blood

_____10. Substance that provokes the immune system

_____11. Type of white blood cell that responds to infectious agents

_____12. White blood cell

TERMS

a. Albumin

b. Antigen

c. Coagulation

d. Erythrocyte

e. Erythropoetin

f. Ferritin

g. Hemoglobin

h. Leukocyte

i. Leukopenia

j. Neutrophil

k. Plasma

l. Platelet

PRONUNCIATIONS

Erythrocyte (e-RITH-roh-siet)

Erythropoiesis (e-RITH-roh-poy-EE-sis)

Erythropoietin (e-RITH-roh-POY-eh-tin)

Fibrinolytic (fie-brin-oh-LIT-ik)

Hematopoiesis (HEE-mat-oh-poy-EE-sis)

Leukocytosis (LOO-ko-sie-TOH-sis)

Leukopenia (LOO-koh-PEE-nee-ah)

Macrocyte (MAK-roh-siet)

Macrophage (MAK-roh-foj)

Megakaryocyte (meg-ah-KARE-YO-siet)

Phagocytosis (FA-goh-sye-TOH-sis)

Polymorphonuclear (POL-ee-mor-foh-NOO-klee-er)

Reticulocyte (re-TIK-yoo-loh-siet)

True or False

For additional study, try to change the false statements to make them true.

_____1. A lymphocyte is a red blood cell.

_____2. A reticulocyte is a red blood cell.

_____3. Hemoglobin is inside the red blood cells.

_____4. The amount of iron needed to avoid anemia is about the same for most people unless they have an unusual disease state.

_____5. Aspirin interferes with platelets and decreases thrombus (clot) formation.

_____6. Doctors order hemoglobin levels for patients to determine the cause and treatment options for anemia.

_____7. White blood cells usually decrease in number when a patient has a bacterial infection.

_____8. A high level of eosinophils may indicate an allergic reaction.

_____9. Smokers tend to have lower levels of hemoglobin than nonsmokers.

_____10. Unwanted or unnecessary thrombus formation can result in stroke.

Short Answer

1. What are the components of blood?

2. What is the primary role of iron in the hematologic system? What happens if a person does not have enough iron?

3. What are the three important processes that make up hemostasis?

4. Name the clotting factors that are dependent on vitamin K. Which medication depends on interfering with vitamin K as its mechanism of action?

5. Describe the role of white blood cells in fighting infection.

CHAPTER 25

Disorders of the Hematologic System

LEARNING OBJECTIVES

After completing this chapter, you should be able to

1. List the different types of anemia
2. Describe the presentation and laboratory abnormalities associated with the different types of anemia
3. State the therapies used to treat each type of anemia
4. Explain/list the factors that cause clot formation and the most common sites of clot formation
5. Describe acute and chronic treatment of clots
6. Explain the therapeutic effects, most common side effects, and adverse reactions of anticoagulant medications
7. State brand and generic names of anticoagulant medications along with routes of administration, dosage forms, and available doses

Matching I

*Match each brand name injected anemia medication with its generic name. For additional study, note whether the treatment is an iron supplement (**I**) or an erythropoetin-stimulating agent (**ESA**).*

Brand Names	Generic Names	I or ESA
1. Aranesp		
2. DexFerrum		
3. Epogen		
4. Feraheme		
5. Ferrlecit		
6. INFeD		
7. Procrit		
8. Venofer		

GENERIC NAMES

a. darbepoetin alfa

b. epoetin alfa

c. ferumoxytol

d. iron dextran

e. iron sucrose

f. sodium ferric gluconate

PRONUNCIATIONS

Agranulocytosis (ay-GRAN-yoo-loh-sie-TOH-sis)

Anti-coagulants (an-tee-koh-AG-yoo-lunts)

Cerebrovascular (ser-ee-broh-VASK-yoo-lar)

Embolus (EM-boh-lus)

Endocarditis (EN-doh-kard-IE-tis)

Endothelial (en-doh-THEE-lee-al)

Ferritin (FAYR-uh-tin)

Haptoglobin (hap-toh-GLOH-bin)

Hematocrit (hee-MAT-o-krit)

Hemoglobin (HEE-muh-gloh-bin)

Hemolytic (HEE-moh-LIT-ik)

Hypercoagulability (hie-per-ko-AG-yoo-luh-BIL-it-ee)

Lactate dehydrogenase (LAK-tayt dee-hie-DROJ-en-ayss)

Myelosuppressive (MY-uh-loh-suh-PRES-iv)

Neutropenia (noo-troh-PEE-nee-uh)

Osteomyelitis (OS-tee-o-my-el-EYE-tis)

Pernicious (per-NISH-us)

Prophylaxis (proh-fuh-LAX-is)

Prothrombin (pro-THROM-bin)

Reticulocyte (re-TIK-yoo-loh-siet)

Stasis (STAY-sis)

Thrombi (THROM-bye)

Thrombocytopenia (throm-boh-sie-toh-PEE-nee-uh)

Thromboplastin (throm-bow-PLAS-tin)

Transferrin (trans-FAYR-in)

Matching II

Match each brand name anticoagulant to its generic name and its class. For additional study, list the route of administration of each medication.

Brand Names	Generic Names	Class	Route of Administration
1. Angiomax			
2. Arixtra			
3. Coumadin			
4. Fragmin			
5. Lovenox			
6. Pradaxa			
7. Xarelto			

GENERIC NAMES

a. bivalirudin

b. dabigatran

c. dalteparin

d. enoxaparin

e. fondaparinux

f. rivaroxaban

g. warfarin

ANTICOAGULANT CLASS

K = Vitamin K antagonist

L = Low molecular weight heparin

T = Thrombin inhibitor

X = Factor Xa inhibitor

True or False

For additional study, try to change the false statements to make them true.

_____1. Macrocytic anemia may be treated with either folic acid or vitamin B12.

_____2. Erythropoetin-stimulating agents such as darbepoetin or epoetin are used to treat anemia associated with chronic kidney disease.

_____3. Patients who have been affected by heparin-induced thrombocytopenia (HIT) should not receive future anticoagulant therapy.

_____4. Low molecular weight heparins (LMWHs) have a shorter duration of action than unfractionated heparin and must be administered more frequently.

_____5. The laboratory value most useful in monitoring and dose adjustment during warfarin therapy is the INR (International Normalized Ratio).

_____6. Dabigatran therapy requires more laboratory tests and dosage adjustments than warfarin therapy.

_____7. Protamine can reverse the anticoagulant actions of heparin but not those of thrombin inhibitors.

_____8. Vitamin K can be administered orally to reverse the anticoagulant actions of warfarin and dabigatran.

_____9. Dabigatran, like warfarin, can be administered orally, but its mechanism of action is unrelated to vitamin K.

_____10. In addition to anticoagulant medication, another therapy for blood clot prevention available from many pharmacies may be TED (thromboembolic disease) stockings.

Short Answer

1. Why is iron supplementation often not the only treatment for iron deficiency anemia?

2. Ferrous fumarate is approximately 33% elemental iron. What daily dose (in mg) of ferrous fumarate would a patient take to get 200 mg of elemental iron?

3. What types of medication may induce neutropenia? What medications are administered to prevent it?

4. Heparin has many uses and indications and several ways it is administered. Name at least two uses and two methods of administration.

5. What special attention and counseling from the pharmacist are important for patients who are taking warfarin?

DRUG MONOGRAPH

Choose one brand-name anticoagulant and complete a drug monograph using the form provided here. (An example of the drug monograph is included in Chapter 1 of this workbook.)

Generic Name _____

Brand Name _____

Manufacturer _____

APPROVED INDICATION(S)

_____
_____
_____
_____

DOSAGE AND ROUTE(S) OF ADMINISTRATION

_____
_____
_____

AVAILABLE DOSAGE FORM(S) STRENGTH(S)

STORAGE/HANDLING CONDITIONS/PROCEDURES

_____
_____

PRECAUTIONS (CONTRAINDICATIONS, DRUG/FOOD INTERACTIONS, PREGNANCY CATEGORY)

_____
_____
_____
_____
_____
_____

COMMON OR SEVERE ADVERSE REACTIONS

_____
_____
_____
_____
_____

INSTRUCTIONS FOR PATIENTS

_____
_____
_____
_____
_____
_____

COST OF THERAPY (DAILY, MONTHLY, FULL COURSE)

_____
_____
_____

OTHER DRUGS IN THIS CLASS

_____
_____
_____

ADDITIONAL MEDICATIONS WITH SAME INDICATION

_____
_____
_____

ADVANTAGES/DISADVANTAGES COMPARED TO DRUGS LISTED ABOVE (CLASS, INDICATION)

_____
_____
_____
_____
_____

CHAPTER 26

Bacterial Infections

LEARNING OBJECTIVES

After completing this chapter, you should be able to

1. Define

   • Bacteria

   • Infection

   • Normal flora

   • Pathogen

   • Resistance

2. Outline the concept of normal flora bacteria and the mechanism behind the development of pathogenicity

3. Describe host defense mechanisms

4. Recognize the types of bacteria and bacterial infections

5. Explain the therapeutic effects of antibiotics and the most common indications for each class

6. Identify factors relevant to antibiotic selection

7. Outline management of patients with bacterial infections, including monitoring for efficacy and safety

PRONUNCIATIONS

α-haemolytic (AL-fuh hee-moh-LIT-ik)

Aerobic (ayr-OH-bik)

Anaerobic (AN-ayr-OH-bik)

Aureus (ARR-ee-us)

Bacillus (buh-SILL-us)

Clostridium (klos-TRID-ee-um)

Coccus (KOK-us)

Coryneform (KOR-nee-form)

Diplococci (DIH-ploh-KOK-eye)

Enterobacteriaceae (EN-ter-oh-bak-teer-ee –AY-see-ee)

Enterococci (EN-ter-oh-KOK-ie)

Escherichia coli (ess-er-IK-ee-uh KOH-lye)

Genus (JEE-nuss)

Immunodeficiency (im-YOO-noh-dee-FISH-en-see)

Immunoglobulins (im-YOO-noh-GLOB-yuh-linz)

Immunosuppression (im-YOO-noh-suh-PRESH-un)

Lactobacilli (LAK-toh-buh-SILL-ie)

Leukocytosis (loo-koh-sye-TOH-sis)

Listeria monocytogenes (liss-TEER-ee-uh mon-oh-sye-TOJ-en-eez)

Morphology (mor-FOL-oh-jee)

Mycobacteria (MYE-koh-bak-TEER-ee-ah)

Neisseria (neis-se-ri-a)

Pathogens (PATH-oh-jenz)

Pseudomonas (soo-doh-MOH-nas)

Salmonella (sal-mo-NEL-uh)

Shigella (shih-GEL-uh)

Spirillum (spih-RIL-um)

Staphylococcus (STAFF-ih-loh-KOK-us)

Streptococci (STREP-toh-kok-eye)

Yersinia (yer-SIN-ee-uh)

Matching I

Match each brand name beta lactam antibiotic to its generic name and route of administration. For additional study, list the class to which each belongs.

Brand Names	Generic Names	Routes	Class
1. Augmentin			
2. Azactam			
3. Bactocill			
4. Bicillin LA			
5. Cedax			
6. Ceftin			
7. Claforan			
8. Doribax			
9. Fortaz			
10. Invanz			
11. Keflex			
12. Mefoxin			
13. Merrem			
14. Moxatag			
15. Nallpen			
16. Primaxin			
17. Rocephin			
18. Spectracef			
19. Suprax			
20. Tazicef			
21. Teflaro			
22. Timentin			
23. Unasyn			
24. Zinacef			
25. Zosyn			

GENERIC NAMES

a. amoxicillin
b. amoxicillin/clavulanate
c. ampicillin/sulbactam
d. aztreonam
e. cefditoren
f. cefixime
g. cefotaxime
h. cefoxitin
i. ceftaroline
j. ceftazidime
k. ceftibuten
l. ceftriaxone

m. cefuroxime
n. cephalexin
o. doripenem
p. ertapenem
q. imipenem/cilastatin
r. meropenem
s. nafcillin
t. oxacillin
u. penicillin G benzathine
v. piperacillin/tazobactam
w. ticarcillin/clavulanate

ROUTES

X = Oral   **Z** = Injection

Matching II

Match each brand name to its generic name and class. For additional study, write in the route(s) of administration.

Brand Names	Generic Names	Class	Route of Administration
1. Akne-Mycin			
2. Avelox			
3. Biaxin			
4. Cetraxal			
5. Ciloxan			
6. Cipro			
7. Dificid			
8. E.E.S.			
9. Erythrocin lactobionate			
10. Factive			
11. Ilotycin			
12. Iquix			
13. Levaquin			
14. Noroxin			
15. Ocuflox			
16. PCE			
17. ProQuin XR			
18. Quixin			
19. Zithromax			
20. Zmax			

GENERIC NAMES

a. azithromycin
b. ciprofloxacin
c. clarithromycin
d. erythromycin
e. fidaxomicin

f. gemifloxacin
g. levofloxacin
h. moxifloxacin
i. norfloxacin
j. ofloxacin

CLASS

M = Macrolide
Q = Fluoroquinolone

Matching III

Match each brand name antibiotic to its generic name and route of administration. For additional study, list the class to which each belongs.

Brand Names	Generic Names	Route of Administration	Class
1. Bactrim			
2. Bleph-10			
3. Cleocin			
4. Coly-Mycin M			
5. Cubicin			
6. Doryx			
7. Flagyl			
8. Furadantin			
9. Macrobid			
10. Minocin			
11. Myambutol			
12. Rifadin			
13. Septra			
14. Seromycin			
15. Solodyn			
16. Synercid			
17. Tygacil			
18. Vibramycin			
19. Xifaxan			
20. Zyvox			

GENERIC NAMES

a. clindamycin

b. colistimethate

c. co-trimoxazole

d. cycloserine

e. daptomycin

f. doxycycline

g. ethambutol

h. linezolid

i. metronidazole

j. minocycline

k. nitrofurantoin

l. quinupristin/dalfopristin

m. rifampin

n. rifamycin

o. sulfacetamide

p. tigecycline

ROUTES

X = Oral

Y = Ophthalmic

Z = Injection

XZ = Oral and injection

True or False

For additional study, try to change the false statements to make them true.

_____1. All bacteria are considered infections when they grow and reside in the human body.

_____2. Nosocomial is a term that refers to upper respiratory tract infections.

_____3. Infections should be treated with the narrowest-spectrum agent to which the causative bacteria are susceptible.

_____4. Reserving broad-spectrum antibiotics for use only when other treatments will not cover the infection promotes development of antibiotic-resistant bacteria.

_____5. Anti-staphylococcal penicillins are effective against gram positive bacteria that produce beta-lactamase, but they are ineffective against gram negative bacteria.

_____6. Cephalosporins are a good type of antibiotic to use for patients who have had a serious or life-threatening allergic reaction to a penicillin.

_____7. Fluoroquinolone antibiotics like ciprofloxacin cover many types of organisms and can be given by many routes of administration related to the location of an infection.

_____8. Patients with allergies to the sulfonamide antibiotics may also be allergic to drugs in other classes, such as the thiazide diuretics or some agents used for diabetes.

_____9. Linezolid is a drug that is effective against many resistant gram positive organisms, but it must be given intravenously because it is not available as an oral formulation and is relatively expensive.

_____10. Combinations of antibiotics may be more effective against some infections and also reduce the chances of bacterial resistance.

Short Answer

1. What is the purpose of obtaining cultures from infected patients, and what determinations can be made from these cultures?

2. What is meant by the term susceptibility, and how does this apply to the choice of antibiotic to treat an infection?

4. What are the most common side effects and adverse reactions associated with penicillin antibiotics? How do they compare with the most common side effects and adverse reactions with cephalosporins and fluoro-quinolones?

3. Why is it said that aminoglycoside antibiotics have a narrow therapeutic window? What monitoring is necessary because of this?

5. What is empiric antibiotic therapy? Give an example of such therapy for a suspected gram positive skin infection.

DRUG MONOGRAPH

Choose one brand-name cephalosporin antibiotic and complete a drug monograph using the form provided here. (An example of the drug monograph is included in Chapter 1 of this workbook.)

Generic Name _____

Brand Name _____

Manufacturer _____

APPROVED INDICATION(S)

_____

_____

_____

_____

DOSAGE AND ROUTE(S) OF ADMINISTRATION

_____

_____

_____

AVAILABLE DOSAGE FORM(S) STRENGTH(S)

STORAGE/HANDLING CONDITIONS/PROCEDURES

_____

_____

_____

PRECAUTIONS (CONTRAINDICATIONS, DRUG/FOOD INTERACTIONS, PREGNANCY CATEGORY)

_____

_____

_____

_____

_____

COMMON OR SEVERE ADVERSE REACTIONS

_____

_____

_____

_____

INSTRUCTIONS FOR PATIENTS

_____

_____

_____

_____

COST OF THERAPY (DAILY, MONTHLY, FULL COURSE)

_____

_____

_____

OTHER DRUGS IN THIS CLASS

_____

_____

ADDITIONAL MEDICATIONS WITH SAME INDICATION

_____

_____

_____

ADVANTAGES/DISADVANTAGES COMPARED TO DRUGS LISTED ABOVE (CLASS, INDICATION)

_____

_____

_____

_____

_____

CHAPTER 27

Viral Infections

LEARNING OBJECTIVES

After completing this chapter, you should be able to

1. Define the following:
   - AIDS
   - DNA
   - RNA
   - Virus

2. Describe common types of viral infections

3. Differentiate between viral infections treated with antiviral therapy and those whose treatment is restricted to supportive care

4. Describe the different types of antiviral medications and the targets of action of each

5. List major adverse effects, cautions, and drug interactions for antiviral medications

PRONUNCIATIONS

Adenopathy (ad-en-OP-uh-thee)

Adenoviruses (AD-eh-noh-VIE-rus-ez)

Cytomegalovirus (sie-toh-MEG-uh-loh-VIE-rus)

Entero viruses (EN-ter-oh-VIE-rus-ez)

Epstein-Barr (EP-steen BAR)

Herpes (HER-peez)

Interferons (in ter FEER onz)

Keratoconjunctivitis (KAYR-uh-toh-kun-junk-tih-VIE-tis)

Microbicide (mie-KROH-bi-sied)

Oncogenic (on-koh-JEN-ik)

Replicate (REH-pli-kayt)

Rhinoviruses (RIE-noh-VIE-rus-ez)

Syncytial (sin-SISH-ul)

Vesicles (VES-ih-kulz)

Matching I

Match each brand name antiviral preparation to its generic name and list the type of viral infection(s) for which it is used. For additional study, list the route of administration for each.

Brand Names	Generic Names	Indication(s)	Route of Administration
1. Baraclude			
2. Copegus			
3. Cytovene			
4. Famvir			
5. Flumadine			
6. Hepsera			
7. Infergen			
8. Intron A			
9. Pegasys			
10. PegIntron			
11. Rebetol			
12. Relenza			
13. Sylatron			
14. Tamiflu			
15. Valcyte			
16. Valtrex			
17. Virazole			
18. Vistide			
19. Zirgan			
20. Zovirax			

GENERIC NAMES

a. acyclovir
b. adefovir
c. cidofovir
d. entecavir
e. famciclovir
f. ganciclovir
g. interferon alfa-2b
h. interferon alfacon-1
i. oseltamivir
j. peginterferon alfa-2a
k. peginterferon alfa-2b
l. ribavirin
m. rimantadine
n. valacyclovir
o. valganciclovir
p. zanamivir

INDICATIONS

CMV = Cytomegalovirus
HBV = Hepatitis B
HCV = Hepatitis C
HSV = Herpes viruses
RSV = Respiratory syncytial virus

Influenza A
Influenza B

Matching II

Match each brand name antiretroviral agent (all used for HIV) with its generic name and mechanism of action.

Brand Names	Generic Names	Mechanism of Action
1. Aptivus		
2. Crixivan		
3. Edurant		
4. Emtriva		
5. Epivir		
6. Fuzeon		
7. Intelence		
8. Invirase		
9. Lexiva		
10. Norvir		
11. Prezista		
12. Rescriptor		
13. Retrovir		
14. Reyataz		
15. Sustiva		
16. Videx		
17. Viracept		
18. Viramune		
19. Zerit		
20. Ziagen		

GENERIC NAMES

a. abacavir
b. atazanavir
c. darunavir
d. delavirdine
e. didanosine
f. efavirenz
g. emtricitabine
h. enfuvirtide
i. etravirine
j. fosamprenavir
k. indinavir
l. lamivudine
m. nelfinavir
n. nevirapine
o. rilpivirine
p. ritonavir
q. saquinavir
r. stavudine
s. tipranavir
t. zidovudine

MECHANISMS OF ACTION

Entry Inhibitor
NNRTI = Non-nucleoside reverse transcriptase inhibitor
NRTI = Nucleoside reverse transcriptase inhibitor
PI = Protease inhibitor

True or False

For additional study, try to change the false statements to make them true.

_____1. Viruses are infectious agents but are not living organisms.

_____2. Enteroviruses affect mainly the upper respiratory tract.

_____3. Herpesvirus infections can be cured by treatment with appropriate antiviral medications.

_____4. There is currently no recommended drug treatment for hepatitis A.

_____5. All viral infections can and should be treated with antiviral medications.

_____6. Neuraminidase inhibitors such as oseltamivir (Tamiflu) are effective against influenza if treatment is begun within 5 days of the onset of symptoms.

_____7. Antiviral interferons may cause flu-like symptoms in patients who are treated with them.

_____8. Some antiviral medications such as zidovudine and cidofovir must be prepared using the same kinds of precautions as cancer chemotherapy (biological safety cabinet, special gloves, etc.) to protect pharmacy personnel from accidental exposure.

_____9. Additional antivirals are not added to therapy with protease inhibitors for HIV to reduce the development of resistant strains.

_____10. Postexposure prophylaxis (PEP) is a regimen of two or three antiretroviral medications from at least two different drug classes that is administered to individuals who have been (or may have been) exposed to HIV.

Short Answer

1. Describe three places in the viral infection cycle where currently available antiviral medications act and give an example of each.

2. What common precaution is emphasized in medication guides for patients taking antivirals for hepatitis, and why?

3. What classes of antiviral medications are currently indicated only for the treatment of influenza? How are they administered?

4. Name at least three medications for CMV (cytomegalovirus) eye infections that are not always placed directly into the eye for treatment, and describe how they are administered.

5. What factors complicate antiretroviral treatment regimens for HIV-infected patients?

DRUG MONOGRAPH

Choose one brand name combination antiretroviral product and complete a drug monograph using the form here. (An example of the drug monograph is included in Chapter 1 of this workbook.)

Generic Name _____

Brand Name _____

Manufacturer _____

APPROVED INDICATION(S)

_____

_____

_____

_____

DOSAGE AND ROUTE(S) OF ADMINISTRATION

_____

_____

_____

AVAILABLE DOSAGE FORM(S) STRENGTH(S)

STORAGE/HANDLING CONDITIONS/PROCEDURES

_____

_____

_____

PRECAUTIONS (CONTRAINDICATIONS, DRUG/FOOD INTERACTIONS, PREGNANCY CATEGORY)

_____

_____

_____

_____

_____

COMMON OR SEVERE ADVERSE REACTIONS

_____

_____

_____

_____

_____

INSTRUCTIONS FOR PATIENTS

_____

_____

_____

_____

COST OF THERAPY (DAILY, MONTHLY, FULL COURSE)

_____

_____

_____

OTHER DRUGS IN THIS CLASS

_____

_____

_____

ADDITIONAL MEDICATIONS WITH SAME INDICATION

_____

_____

_____

_____

ADVANTAGES/DISADVANTAGES COMPARED TO DRUGS LISTED ABOVE (CLASS, INDICATION)

_____

_____

_____

_____

CHAPTER 28

Fungal Infections

LEARNING OBJECTIVES

After completing this chapter, you should be able to

1. Compare and contrast the mechanisms of action of various classes of antifungal agents
2. Describe side effects commonly associated with each of the antifungal classes
3. Describe the drug interaction potential for each class of antifungals
4. List the formulations available for each antifungal agent

Matching

Match each brand name product to the generic antifungal it contains and its route(s) of administration. For additional study, list the available dosage forms of the product.

Brand Names	Generic Names	Route of Administration	Dosage Form(s)
1. Abelcet			
2. Ambisome			
3. Amphotec			
4. Cancidas			
5. Diflucan			
6. Eraxis			
7. Monistat			
8. Mycamine			
9. Noxafil			
10. Sporanox			
11. Terbinex			
12. Vfend			

GENERIC NAMES

a. amphotericin B
b. anidulafungin
c. caspofungin
d. fluconazole
e. itraconazole
f. micafungin
g. miconazole
h. posaconazole
i. terbinafine
j. voriconazole

ROUTES

PO = Oral   **IV =** Intravenous   **V =** Vaginal

PRONUNCIATIONS

Aspergillosis (ass-per-jil-OH-sis)
Candida (KAN-dee-duh)
Dermatophyte (der-MAT-oh-fite)
Eukaryotic (yoo-KAYR-ee-OT-ik)
Fungi (FUN-jie)
Fungus (FUN-gus)

True or False

For additional study, try to change the false statements to make them true.

_____1. A fungal cell resembles a bacterial cell because it has a membrane-bound nucleus and organelles.

_____2. Fungal cells, like bacterial cells, have a cell wall, making them susceptible to the same antibiotic medications used to treat bacterial infections.

_____3. The terms mold and yeast may be applied to the kinds of organisms that cause fungal infections.

_____4. Lipid-based antifungal preparations are classified as suspensions, but they contain no solid particulate matter and can be administered intravenously.

_____5. Azole antifungals, such as itraconazole, have many drug interactions because they interfere with kidney excretion of several medications.

_____6. Both voriconazole and fluconazole may be used in the treatment of Aspergillus fungal infections.

_____7. Echinocandin antifungals (micafungin, caspofungin, anidulafungin) must be administered only by the intravenous route.

_____8. For fungal infections of the toenails, terbinafine is always applied topically directly to the nailbed.

_____9. Griseofulvin is administered orally and is commonly used to treat children who have fungal infections of the scalp.

_____10. Coccidioidomycosis is a fungal infection that is seldom treated with medication unless the patient is immunocompromised.

Short Answer

1. What is an opportunistic pathogen? How does this description relate to the types of patients most likely to be treated for serious fungal infections?

2. Discuss the interchangeability, differences, and similarities of the available lipid-based amphotericin B preparations.

3. Why is nystatin not used to treat systemic fungal infections? How does this fact relate to the uses it has and to its side effect profile?

4. How is fluconazole administered? For what kinds of infections is it used, and what are its limitations?

5. What is meant by endemic infections? What are the most common endemic fungal infections in the United States, and how do they spread?

DRUG MONOGRAPH

Choose one brand name antifungal product and complete a drug monograph using the form provided here. (An example of the drug monograph is included in Chapter 1 of this workbook.)

Generic Name _____

Brand Name _____

Manufacturer _____

APPROVED INDICATION(S)

_____
_____
_____
_____

DOSAGE AND ROUTE(S) OF ADMINISTRATION

_____
_____
_____

AVAILABLE DOSAGE FORM(S) STRENGTH(S)

STORAGE/HANDLING CONDITIONS/PROCEDURES

_____
_____
_____

PRECAUTIONS (CONTRAINDICATIONS, DRUG/FOOD INTERACTIONS, PREGNANCY CATEGORY)

_____
_____
_____
_____
_____

COMMON OR SEVERE ADVERSE REACTIONS

_____
_____
_____
_____
_____
_____
_____

INSTRUCTIONS FOR PATIENTS

_____
_____
_____
_____
_____

COST OF THERAPY (DAILY, MONTHLY, FULL COURSE)

_____
_____
_____

OTHER DRUGS IN THIS CLASS

_____
_____
_____

ADDITIONAL MEDICATIONS WITH SAME INDICATION

_____
_____
_____
_____

ADVANTAGES/DISADVANTAGES COMPARED TO DRUGS LISTED ABOVE (CLASS, INDICATION)

_____
_____
_____
_____
_____

CHAPTER 29

Immunobiologics

LEARNING OBJECTIVES

After completing this chapter, you should be able to

1. Describe the immune system and the types of immunity
2. Discuss the importance of disease prevention to public health and how pharmacy personnel can contribute
3. Describe the different types of immunizations
4. List recommended immunizations for various populations and purposes
5. Discuss the uses of monoclonal antibodies
6. Discuss the therapeutic uses of immunosuppression and list agents used for this purpose

PRONUNCIATIONS

Antibodies (AN-ti-bod-eez)

Antigens (ANT-ih-jenz)

Immune globulin (im-YOON GLOB-yoo-lin)

Immunization (im-yoo-niz-AY-shun)

Immunocompromise (im-YOON-oh-KOM-proh-mize)

Immunosuppressives (im-YOON-oh-sup-res-ivz)

Innate (in-AYT)

Live-attenuated (LIEV uh-TEN-yoo-ay-ted)

Lymphatic (lim-FAT-ik)

Rejection (ree-JEK-shun)

Toxoid (TOK-soyd)

Vaccination (VAK-sin-AY-shun)

Vaccine (VAK-seen)

Matching I

Match each brand name vaccine or toxoid to the type of infection(s) it prevents. For additional study, identify the ones that are administered by routes other than intramuscular (IM).

Brand Names	Type of Infection(s)	Routes Other Than IM
1. Adacel		
2. BCG		
3. Boostrix		
4. Engerix-B		
5. Fluarix		
6. FluMist		
7. Fluzone		
8. Gardasil		
9. Havrix		
10. Hiberix		
11. Menactra		
12. Menveo		
13. M-M-R II		
14. Pediarix		
15. Prevnar 13		
16. Recombivax-HB		
17. Rotarix		
18. Vaqta		
19. Varivax		
20. Zostavax		

INFECTIONS

a. Diphtheria
b. *H. influenza* B
c. Hepatitis A
d. Hepatitis B
e. Herpes zoster
f. Human papilloma virus
g. Influenza
h. Measles
i. Meningococcus

j. Mumps
k. Pertussis
l. Poliovirus
m. Rotavirus
n. Rubella
o. *Streptococcus pneumoniae* (pneumococcus)
p. Tetanus
q. Tuberculosis
r. Varicella

Matching II

Match each brand name immunosuppressive agent to its generic name. For additional study, look up each product to determine its route(s) of administration

Brand Names	Generic Names	Route of Administration
1. Afinitor		
2. Atgam		
3. CellCept		
4. Gengraf		
5. Hecoria		
6. Imuran		
7. Myfortic		
8. Neoral		
9. Nulojix		
10. Prograf		
11. Rapamune		
12. Sandimmune		
13. Thymoglobulin		
14. Zortress		

GENERIC NAMES

a. antithymocyte globulin (equine)
b. antithymocyte globulin (rabbit)
c. azathioprine
d. belatacept
e. cyclosporine
f. everolimus
g. mycophenolate
h. sirolimus
i. tacrolimus

True or False

For additional study, try to change the false statements to make them true.

_____1. Resistance to an infection after exposure to the pathogen that causes it, either after recovering from an infection or by receiving a vaccination, is termed active immunity.

_____2. The immunity acquired after receiving an immune globulin is immediate and long-lasting or even lifelong.

_____3. Some vaccines labeled for children should not be administered to adults.

_____4. All vaccines are administered by injection.

_____5. Tetanus and influenza vaccinations should be repeated every 10 years.

_____6.   Vaccination against herpes zoster is not recommended for children.

_____7.   Organ transplant patients receive immunosuppressive medications to avoid infection after their transplant surgery.

_____8.   Mycophenolate tablets can be chewed or dissolved if the patient has trouble swallowing them whole.

_____9.   There are several different cyclosporine preparations, but they are not considered eligible for automatic generic substitution.

_____10. Pharmacy technicians who prepare or dispense immunosuppressants should take the same precautions that they would with hazardous cancer chemotherapy agents.

Short Answer

1. What is an immune globulin? What effect does administration of an immune globulin preparation have on the immune system of a patient?

2. Why is proper storage and handling so important for immunizations? What important duties do pharmacy technicians have with respect to these pharmaceuticals?

3. How can patients be immunized to certain diseases by administration of pharmaceuticals?

4. What is post-exposure prophylaxis? Give an example of the use of an immunobiologic preparation for this purpose.

5. Why does cyclosporine have a large number of drug interactions? What adverse effects could occur as a result of an interaction between cyclosporine and another medication?

DRUG MONOGRAPH

Choose one brand name immune globulin product and complete a drug monograph using the form provided here. (An example of the drug monograph is included in Chapter 1 of this workbook.)

Generic Name _____

Brand Name _____

Manufacturer _____

APPROVED INDICATION(S)

_____
_____
_____
_____

DOSAGE AND ROUTE(S) OF ADMINISTRATION

_____
_____
_____

AVAILABLE DOSAGE FORM(S) STRENGTH(S)

_____
_____
_____

STORAGE/HANDLING CONDITIONS/PROCEDURES

_____
_____
_____

PRECAUTIONS (CONTRAINDICATIONS, DRUG/FOOD INTERACTIONS, PREGNANCY CATEGORY)

_____
_____
_____
_____
_____

COMMON OR SEVERE ADVERSE REACTIONS

_____
_____
_____
_____
_____

INSTRUCTIONS FOR PATIENTS

_____
_____
_____
_____

COST OF THERAPY (DAILY, MONTHLY, FULL COURSE)

_____
_____
_____

OTHER DRUGS IN THIS CLASS

_____
_____
_____

ADDITIONAL MEDICATIONS WITH SAME INDICATION

_____
_____
_____

ADVANTAGES/DISADVANTAGES COMPARED TO DRUGS LISTED ABOVE (CLASS, INDICATION)

_____
_____
_____
_____
_____

CHAPTER 30

Cancer

LEARNING OBJECTIVES

After completing this chapter, you should be able to

1. List the classes of agents used to treat cancer, including their place in therapy, and give examples of each
2. Recognize the side effects of different types of chemotherapeutic agents
3. Define medical terms used in chemotherapy management
4. List the risk factors for chemotherapy-related nausea and vomiting and discuss medications used in its treatment
5. Recognize look-alike/sound-alike medications used in treating the oncology patient

PRONUNCIATIONS

Adjuvant (AJ-uv-ent)

Alkylating agent (AL-kuh-LAY-ting AY-jent)

Alopecia (al-uh-PEE-shuh)

Anaphylaxis (AN-uh-fil-AK-sis)

Anthracycline (an-thruh-SYE-kleen)

Antimetabolite (an-TYE-meh-TAB-oh-lite)

Antimitotics (an-tee-mye-TOT-iks)

Antineoplastic (an-tye-nee-oh-PLAS-tik)

Apoptosis (A-pop-TOH-sis)

Aromatase inhibitors (uh-ROH-muh-tayz in-HIH-bih-terz)

Benign (bee-NINE)

Camptothecins (kam-toh-THEE-sinz)

Cancer (KAN-ser)

Carcinoid (KAR-sin-oid)

Carcinoma (kar-sin-OH-muh)

Cardiotoxicity (KAR-dee-oh-tok-SIS-it-ee)

Chemotherapy (kee-moh-THAYR-up-ee)

Cytokines (SY-toh-kines)

Cytoprotective (SYE-toh-proh-TEK-tiv)

Cytotoxic (sye-toh-TOKS-ik)

Emetogenic (eh-MET-oh-JEN-ik)

Extravasation (eks-TRAV-uh-ZAY-shun)

Folate (FOH-layt)

Hemorrhagic cystitis (hem-eh-RAJ-ik sis-TYE-tis)

Hormonal (hor-MOHN-ul)

Hydrated (HYE-dray-ted)

Interferons (in-ter-FEER-onz)

Interleukins (in-ter-LOO-kinz)

Leukemia (loo-KEE-mee-uh)

Continued on next page

PRONUNCIATIONS (cont'd)

Malignancies (muh-LIG-nun-seez)

Malignant (muh-LIG-nunt)

Metastases (meh-TAS-tus-eez)

Metastasis (meh-TAS-tuh-sis)

Metastasize (meh-TAS-tuh-size)

Metastatic (meh-tuh-STAT-ik)

Mucositis (myoo-koh-SYE-tis)

Mutation (myoo-TAY-shun)

Myelosuppression (MYE-uh-loh-suh-PRESH-un)

Neoplasm (NEE-oh-PLAZ-um)

Neuroendocrine (nyoor-oh-EN-doh-krin)

Neutropenia (noo-troh-PEE-nee-uh)

Oncologist (on-KOL-oh-jist)

Oncology (on-KOL-oh-jee)

Palliative (PAL-ee-uh-tiv)

Peripheral (per-IF-er-ul) neuropathy (nyer-OP-uth-ee)

Podophyllotoxin (poh-DOF-il-oh-TOK-sin)

Proliferate (proh-LIF-er-ayt)

Sarcoma (sar-KOH-muh)

Tumor (TOO-mer)

Vesicants (VEH-sih-kantz)

Matching I

Match each brand name cancer chemotherapy to its generic name. For additional study, list the type(s) of cancer it is used to treat.

Brand Names	Generic Names	Type of Cancer
1. Abraxane		
2. Adriamycin		
3. Alimta		
4. Arimidex		
5. Camptosar		
6. Casodex		
7. Doxil		
8. Eligard		
9. Eloxatin		
10. Femara		
11. Gemzar		
12. Hydrea		
13. Ifex		
14. Leukeran		
15. Lupron		
16. Myleran		
17. Navelbine		
18. Taxotere		
19. Xeloda		
20. Zoladex		

GENERIC NAMES

a. anastrozole

b. bicalutamide

c. busulfan

d. capecitabine

e. chlorambucil

f. docetaxel

g. doxorubicin

h. doxorubicin liposomal

i. gemcitabine

j. goserelin

k. hydroxyurea

l. ifosfamide

m. irinotecan

n. letrozole

o. leuprolide

p. oxaliplatin

q. paclitaxel

r. pemetrexed

s. vinorelbine

Matching II

*Match each brand name biologic therapy to its generic name and route of administration (**PO** or **IV**). For additional study, list the type(s) of cancer each is used to treat.*

Brand Names	Generic Names	Route of Administration	Type of Cancer
1. Avastin			
2. Erbitux			
3. Gleevec			
4. Herceptin			
5. Iressa			
6. Proleukin			
7. Rituxan			
8. Sutent			
9. Tarceva			
10. Yervoy			

GENERIC NAMES

a. aldesleukin

b. bevacizumab

c. cetuximab

d. erlotinib

e. gefitinib

f. imatinib

g. ipilimumab

h. rituximab

i. sunitinib

j. trastuzumab

True or False

For additional study, try to change the false statements to make them true.

_____1. Antineoplastic chemotherapy refers to medication used to treat cancer.

_____2. Emetogenic potential refers to the tendency of a medication to interfere with production of blood cells and platelets.

_____3. Ifosfamide chemotherapy must always be accompanied by treatment with mesna.

_____4. Vitamin supplements containing folic acid should be avoided by patients taking pemetrexed.

_____5. It is common for patients to receive large volumes of IV fluids in conjunction with cyclophosphamide doses.

_____6. Patients taking methotrexate should be advised to avoid excess sun exposure.

_____7. Vinca alkaloids for the treatment of central nervous system cancers are usually administered intrathecally.

_____8. Hormonal therapies like aromatase inhibitors are used only in the treatment of life-threatening tumors.

_____9. Chemotherapies in liposomal or protein-bound forms are generically equivalent to other dosage forms and may be substituted without consultation depending on the pharmacy's inventory.

_____10. Anthracycline antineoplastics can cause a red or orange discoloration in the urine of patients who are being treated with them.

Short Answer

1. How is body surface area determined, and what units are used to express this measurement? Why is BSA used for dosing cancer chemotherapy?

2. What are biologic response modifiers? What is the role of agents in this class in the treatment of cancer?

3. What is a cytoprotective agent? Give an example of the use of such a medication as part of a cancer chemotherapy treatment.

4. What is meant by a cancer chemotherapy regimen? Why are antineoplastic medications ordered in combinations?

5. What is myelosuppression? Why is it considered a serious side effect of antineoplastic therapy?

DRUG MONOGRAPH

Choose one brand name cancer treatment agent and complete a drug monograph using the form provided here. (An example of the drug monograph is included in Chapter 1 of this workbook.)

Generic Name _____

Brand Name _____

Manufacturer _____

APPROVED INDICATION(S)

_____

_____

_____

DOSAGE AND ROUTE(S) OF ADMINISTRATION

_____

_____

_____

AVAILABLE DOSAGE FORM(S) STRENGTH(S)

STORAGE/HANDLING CONDITIONS/PROCEDURES

_____

_____

PRECAUTIONS (CONTRAINDICATIONS, DRUG/FOOD INTERACTIONS, PREGNANCY CATEGORY)

_____

_____

_____

_____

COMMON OR SEVERE ADVERSE REACTIONS

_____

_____

_____

_____

_____

_____

INSTRUCTIONS FOR PATIENTS

_____

_____

_____

_____

COST OF THERAPY (DAILY, MONTHLY, FULL COURSE)

_____

_____

_____

OTHER DRUGS IN THIS CLASS

_____

_____

_____

ADDITIONAL MEDICATIONS WITH SAME INDICATION

_____

_____

_____

ADVANTAGES/DISADVANTAGES COMPARED TO DRUGS LISTED ABOVE (CLASS, INDICATION)

_____

_____

_____

_____

CHAPTER 31

Overview of the Skin and Topical Dosage Forms

LEARNING OBJECTIVES

After completing this chapter, you should be able to

1. Describe the skin as an organ system

    a. List the three functionally distinct regions of the skin and describe their function

    b. Describe the roles of keratinocytes, melanocytes, and Langerhans cells as components of the epidermis

    c. Define mast cell

    d. Identify the skin appendages that are located in the dermis

    e. Define adipose tissue

2. Explain how changes in skin thickness, integrity, hydration, and age can alter topical drug absorption

3. Describe how the vehicle in a topical formulation can influence the absorption of the active drug

4. Name and describe two types of transdermal preparations

PRONUNCIATIONS

Epidermis (ep-ee-DER-mis)

Integumentary (in-TEG-yoo-MEN-tuh-ree)

Melanocyte (mel-AN-oh-site)

Stratum corneum (STRAT-um KOR-nee-um)

Topical (TOP-ik-ul)

Transdermal (tranz-DER-mul)

Matching

Match each transdermal patch to its generic ingredient(s). For additional study, write the indication (use) next to each product.

Brand Names	Generic Ingredients	Indication
1. Alora		
2. Androderm		
3. Catapres-TTS		
4. Climara		
5. CombiPatch		
6. Daytrana		
7. Duragesic		
8. Emsam		
9. Estraderm		
10. Exelon		
11. Flector		
12. Habitrol		
13. Lidoderm		
14. Minitran		
15. Nicoderm		
16. Nitro-Dur		
17. Ortho Evra		
18. Oxytrol		
19. Transderm Scōp		
20. Vivelle-Dot		

GENERIC INGREDIENTS

a. clonidine
b. diclofenac
c. estradiol
d. estradiol/norethindrone
e. ethinyl estradiol/norelgestromin
f. fentanyl
g. lidocaine
h. methylphenidate

i. nicotine
j. nitroglycerine
k. oxybutynin
l. rivastigmine
m. scopolamine
n. selegiline
o. testosterone

True or False

For additional study, try to change the false statements to make them true.

_____1. The outermost layer of the skin is the epidermis.

_____2. Topical dusting powders are safe dosage forms with no notable precautions.

_____3. The transdermal route of administration is intended to provide a local effect for medications.

_____4. Some transdermal patches are designed to deliver medication for up to a full week, while others must be changed more frequently.

_____5. OTC products applied to the skin cannot cause drug overdoses.

_____6. Ointments intended for the skin should not be used in the eye.

_____7. Transdermal patches should always be applied to the same spot where the last one was placed.

_____8. Absorption of medications from transdermal patches is not as steady and predictable as it is from dosage forms given orally.

_____9. Most transdermal patches should be removed before patients undergo MRI diagnostic procedures.

_____10. Nitroglycerin patches for angina should be removed 10 to 12 hours before the next one is applied.

Short Answer

1. Distinguish between local and systemic drug actions. Give an example of each.

2. Why are very young children more at risk from adverse systemic effects of medications applied to the skin? What can a pharmacy technician do to help reduce the risk?

3. Name and describe the dosage forms used for medications administered topically.

4. What are the special considerations for the use of transdermal patches, and how can pharmacy technicians assist patients in doing this correctly?

5. Why must transdermal patches never be cut or torn before use?

DRUG MONOGRAPH

*Choose one brand name product from the **Medication Drug Tables** and complete a drug monograph using the form provided here. (An example of the drug monograph is included in Chapter 1 of this workbook.)*

Generic Name _____

Brand Name _____

Manufacturer _____

APPROVED INDICATION(S)

_____

_____

_____

_____

DOSAGE AND ROUTE(S) OF ADMINISTRATION

_____

_____

_____

AVAILABLE DOSAGE FORM(S) STRENGTH(S)

STORAGE/HANDLING CONDITIONS/PROCEDURES

_____

_____

_____

PRECAUTIONS (CONTRAINDICATIONS, DRUG/FOOD INTERACTIONS, PREGNANCY CATEGORY)

_____

_____

_____

_____

_____

COMMON OR SEVERE ADVERSE REACTIONS

_____

_____

_____

_____

_____

_____

INSTRUCTIONS FOR PATIENTS

_____

_____

_____

_____

COST OF THERAPY (DAILY, MONTHLY, FULL COURSE)

_____

_____

_____

OTHER DRUGS IN THIS CLASS

_____

_____

ADDITIONAL MEDICATIONS WITH SAME INDICATION

_____

_____

_____

ADVANTAGES/DISADVANTAGES COMPARED TO DRUGS LISTED ABOVE (CLASS, INDICATION)

_____

_____

_____

_____

_____

_____

CHAPTER 32

Treatment of Dermatologic Disorders

LEARNING OBJECTIVES

After completing this chapter, you should be able to

1. Define the most common dermatologic disorders

2. Explain the disease process (pathophysiology) of each dermatologic disorder

3. Describe nonpharmacologic treatment options for dermatologic disorders

4. State the brand and generic names of the most widely used medications indicated for dermatologic disorders, along with their routes of administration, dosage forms, and available doses

5. Explain the mechanism of action and common adverse effects of prescription and nonprescription agents for the treatment of dermatologic disorders

6. Recognize commonly used treatment regimens for each dermatologic disorder

PRONUNCIATIONS

Astringent (uh-STRIN-jent)

Cellulitis (cel-yoo-LIE-tis)

Comedone (KOH-meh-dohn)

Dermatitis (der-muh-TIE-tis)

Dermatophytosis (dur-mat-oh-FYE-toh-sis)

Emollient (ee-MOL-yunt)

Folliculitis (foh-lik-yoo-LIE-tis)

Impetigo (im-peh-TIE-goh)

Onychomycosis (ON-i-ko-mi-KO-sis)

Psoriasis (sor-IE-uh-sis)

Teratogen (the-RAT-oh-jen)

Tinea (TIN-ee-ah)

Urushiol (yoo-ROO-shee-ol)

Matching I

Match each brand name acne product to its generic name. For additional study, label the ones that can be administered orally.

Brand Names	Generic Names	Oral Administration
1. Aczone		
2. Akne-Mycin		
3. Amnesteem		
4. Avage		
5. Avita		
6. Benzac AC		
7. BenzaShave		
8. Benziq		
9. Brevoxyl		
10. Claravis		
11. ClindaMax		
12. Desquam-X		
13. Differin		
14. Epiduo		
15. Ery-Tab		
16. Evoclin		
17. Pacnex		
18. PanOxyl		
19. Renova		
20. Retin-A		
21. Sotret		
22. Tazorac		
23. Tretin-X		
24. Triaz		
25. Vibramycin		

GENERIC NAMES

a. adapalene

b. benzoyl peroxide

c. benzoyl peroxide+adapalene

d. clindamycin

e. dapsone

f. doxycycline

g. erythromycin

h. isotretinoin

i. tazarotene

j. tretinoin

Matching II

Match each brand name topical corticosteroid to its generic name. For additional study, list the dosage forms (cream, gel, etc.) available.

Brand Names	Generic Names	Dosage Form
1. Aclovate		
2. ApexiCon		
3. Clobex		
4. Cloderm		
5. Cordran		
6. Cormax		
7. Cutivate		
8. DesOwen		
9. Elocon		
10. Halog		
11. Kenalog		
12. Locoid		
13. Luxiq		
14. Olux		
15. Synalar		
16. Temovate		
17. Topicort		
18. Ultravate		
19. Vanos		
20. Westcort		

GENERIC NAMES

a. alclometasone dipropionate

b. betamethasone valerate

c. clobetasol propionate

d. clocortolone pivalate

e. desonide

f. desoximetasone

g. diflorasone diacetate

h. fluocinolone acetonide

i. fluocinonide

j. flurandrenolide

k. fluticasone propionate

l. halcinonide

m. halobetasol propionate

n. hydrocortisone butyrate

o. hydrocortisone valerate

p. mometasone furoate

q. triamcinolone acetonide

Matching III

Match each brand name topical preparation to its generic name. For additional study, list the indication(s) for each product.

Brand Names	Generic Names	Indications
1. Altabax		
2. AmLactin		
3. Aveeno		
4. Bactroban		
5. Balmex		
6. Burow's		
7. Calcitrene		
8. Desitin		
9. Dovonex		
10. Dritho-Creme		
11. Ertaczo		
12. Exelderm		
13. Ionil-T		
14. Lac-Hydrin		
15. Loprox		
16. Lotrimin Ultra		
17. Mentax		
18. Micatin		
19. Neosporin		
20. Nizoral		
21. Oxistat		
22. Penlac		
23. Polysporin		
24. Taclonex		
25. Tinactin		
26. Tucks		
27. Vectical		
28. Xolegel		
29. Zeasorb-AF		
30. Zithranol		

GENERIC NAMES

a. aluminum acetate
b. ammonium lactate
c. anthralin
d. butenafine
e. calcipotriene
f. calcipotriene/betamethasone
g. calcitriol
h. ciclopirox
i. coal tar
j. colloidal oatmeal
k. ketoconazole
l. miconazole
m. mupirocin
n. neomycin/polymyxin/bacitracin
o. oxiconazole
p. polymyxin/bacitracin
q. retapamulin
r. sertaconazole
s. sulconazole
t. tolnaftate
u. witch hazel
v. zinc oxide

True or False

For additional study, try to change the false statements to make them true.

_____1.   While there are many OTC acne treatments, they are seldom effective and should not be recommended.

_____2.   Prescription therapy for psoriasis often involves immunosuppressive agents.

_____3.   Diaper rash is a form of allergic contact dermatitis.

_____4.   The rash from poison ivy is a form of allergic contact dermatitis.

_____5.   Areas of the skin exposed to poison oak should be scrubbed vigorously with an abrasive cleanser to remove the allergen.

_____6.   Oral antibiotics are not used to treat skin infections.

_____7.   Ringworm is a fungal infection and is treated with both oral and topical antifungal medications.

_____8.   Treatment for athlete's foot should be continued only as long as the itching persists.

_____9.   OTC salicylic acid treatment for warts may take up to 12 weeks to work.

_____10. The first-line treatment for lice is an OTC preparation of permethrin.

Short Answer

1. What is the most serious side effect associated with oral isotretinoin therapy for acne? What program has been developed to prevent these effects, and what requirements does it impose on the pharmacy staff?

2. Why is biologic response modifier psoriasis therapy reserved for the treatment of only the most severe cases?

3. What are the two types of contact dermatitis? How do they differ in their causes and treatment?

4. What is the recommended treatment for cold sores?

5. Why is it important for members of the pharmacy staff to understand the implications of various skin conditions?

DRUG MONOGRAPH

*Choose one brand name preparation from **Medication Drug Table 32-8** and complete a drug monograph using the form provided here. (An example of the drug monograph is included in Chapter 1 of this workbook.)*

Generic Name _____

Brand Name _____

Manufacturer _____

APPROVED INDICATION(S)

_____

_____

_____

DOSAGE AND ROUTE(S) OF ADMINISTRATION

_____

_____

_____

AVAILABLE DOSAGE FORM(S) STRENGTH(S)

STORAGE/HANDLING CONDITIONS/PROCEDURES

_____

_____

PRECAUTIONS (CONTRAINDICATIONS, DRUG/FOOD INTERACTIONS, PREGNANCY CATEGORY)

_____

_____

_____

_____

COMMON OR SEVERE ADVERSE REACTIONS

_____

_____

_____

_____

_____

INSTRUCTIONS FOR PATIENTS

_____

_____

_____

_____

_____

COST OF THERAPY (DAILY, MONTHLY, FULL COURSE)

_____

_____

_____

OTHER DRUGS IN THIS CLASS

_____

_____

_____

ADDITIONAL MEDICATIONS WITH SAME INDICATION

_____

_____

_____

_____

ADVANTAGES/DISADVANTAGES COMPARED TO DRUGS LISTED ABOVE (CLASS, INDICATION)

_____

_____

_____

_____

_____

CHAPTER 33

Ophthalmic Medications

LEARNING OBJECTIVES

After completing this chapter, you should be able to

1. Review the anatomy and physiology of the eye

2. Describe glaucoma and the most commonly used treatment approaches

3. Describe the causes and symptoms of conjunctivitis and treatment options

4. Identify common causes of blindness

5. Identify medications used in the eye including their dosage forms, therapeutic effects, most common side effects, and mechanisms of action

Matching I

Match each brand name ophthalmic drop for glaucoma with its generic name. For additional study, write in the class to which each medication belongs.

Brand Names	Generic Names	Class
1. Alphagan		
2. Azopt		
3. Betagan		
4. Betoptic-S		
5. Iopidine		
6. Isopto Carpine		
7. Lumigan		
8. Miostat		
9. Optipranolol		
10. Timoptic		
11. Travatan Z		
12. Trusopt		

GENERIC NAMES

a. apraclonidine

b. betaxolol

c. bimatoprost

d. brimonidine

e. brinzolamide

f. carbachol

g. dorzolamide

h. levobunolol

i. metipranolol

j. pilocarpine

k. timolol

l. travoprost

PRONUNCIATIONS

Aqueous humor (AY-kwee-us HYOO-mer)

Cataract (KAT-ah-rakt)

Conjunctivitis (con-junk-tih-VIE-tis)

Cornea (KOR-nee-ah)

Cycloplegia (sie-kloh-PLEE-juh)

Diplopia (dip-LOH-pee-ah)

Glaucoma (glah-KOH-mah)

Iris (EYE-riss)

Macula (MAK-yoo-luh)

Miosis (mie-OH-siss)

Mydriasis (mid-RIE-uh-siss)

Myopia (mie-OH-pee-uh)

Presbyopia (prez-bee-OH-pee-ah)

Pupil (PYOO-pil)

Retina (RET-na)

Sclera (SKLAYR-uh)

Matching II

Match each brand name eye drop for conjunctivitis with its generic name For additional study, write in the class to which each agent belongs and note which products are available OTC.

Brand Names	Generic Names	Class	OTC
1. Alaway			
2. Alocril			
3. Alomide			
4. AzaSite			
5. Bepreve			
6. Besivance			
7. Bleph-10			
8. Ciloxan			
9. Claritin eye			
10. Elestat			
11. Emadine			
12. Gentak			
13. Iquix			
14. Moxeza			
15. Natacyn			
16. Ocuflox			
17. Optivar			
18. Pataday			
19. Patanol			
20. Tobrex			
21. Vigamox			
22. Viroptic			
23. Zaditor			
24. Zymaxid			
25. Zyrtec itchy eye			

GENERIC NAMES

a.	azelastine	k.	levofloxacin
b.	azithromycin	l.	lodoxamide
c.	bepotastine	m.	moxifloxacin
d.	besifloxacin	n.	natamycin
e.	ciprofloxacin	o.	nedocromil
f.	emedastine	p.	ofloxacin
g.	epinastine	q.	olopatadine
h.	gatifloxacin	r.	sulfacetamide
i.	gentamicin	s.	tobramycin
j.	ketotifen	t.	trifluridine

Matching III

Match each brand name ophthalmic anti-inflammatory to its generic name. For additional study, note whether each preparation is a corticosteroid or a NSAID.

Brand Names	Generic Names	Corticosteroid/ NSAID
1. Acular		
2. Acuvail		
3. Alrex		
4. Durezol		
5. Flarex		
6. FML		
7. Lotemax		
8. Maxidex		
9. Nevanac		
10. Omnipred		
11. Pred Forte		
12. Vexol		

GENERIC NAMES

a.	dexamethasone	e.	loteprednol
b.	difluprednate	f.	nepafenac
c.	fluorometholone	g.	prednisolone
d.	ketorolac	h.	rimexolone

True or False

For additional study, try to change the false statements to make them true.

_____1. Eye drops for glaucoma all work by decreasing intraocular pressure, so it is useless for a patient to have a prescription for more than one at a time.

_____2. OTC ophthalmic decongestants should not be used longer than three consecutive days.

_____3. Treatments for macular degeneration are usually administered as eye drops.

_____4. Brand-name Claritin and Zyrtec are antihistamine drops for the eye that have different active ingredients from the preparations with the same brand names that are given by mouth.

_____5. Patients using ophthalmic antihistamines must be warned that they are likely to cause drowsiness.

_____6. Ophthalmic drops, like intravenous infusions, must be sterile but may be either solutions or suspensions.

_____7. For patients with two eye drops to be administered at the same time, those in solution form should be administered first, followed 5 minutes later by those which are gel-forming drops.

_____8. Contact lenses need not be removed before administration of medicated eye drops.

_____9. Some of the antibiotics in drops for ophthalmic infections have the same active ingredients as those in oral preparations.

_____10. Dry eyes can be treated effectively only with prescription medications prescribed by a physician.

Short Answer

1. Discuss why some ophthalmic drops can be used in the ear, but similar otic drops cannot be used in the eye.

2. Why are ophthalmic suspensions rolled between the hands before administration? Why should shaking them be avoided?

3. What is mydriasis, and why is it helpful during eye examinations? What agents are used to cause it for this purpose, and why are patients who receive them told not to drive themselves home after the exam?

4. Name two classes of agents used in the treatment of glaucoma and describe how each type works.

5. What are the most common side effects of anti-infective eye drops?

DRUG MONOGRAPH

*Choose one brand name agent for the treatment of macular degeneration (see **Medication Table 33-2**) and complete a drug monograph using the form provided here. (An example of the drug monograph is included in Chapter 1 of this workbook.)*

Generic Name _____

Brand Name _____

Manufacturer _____

APPROVED INDICATION(S)

_____

_____

_____

DOSAGE AND ROUTE(S) OF ADMINISTRATION

_____

_____

AVAILABLE DOSAGE FORM(S) STRENGTH(S)

STORAGE/HANDLING CONDITIONS/PROCEDURES

_____

_____

PRECAUTIONS (CONTRAINDICATIONS, DRUG/FOOD INTERACTIONS, PREGNANCY CATEGORY)

_____

_____

_____

_____

COMMON OR SEVERE ADVERSE REACTIONS

_____

_____

_____

_____

_____

INSTRUCTIONS FOR PATIENTS

_____

_____

_____

_____

COST OF THERAPY (DAILY, MONTHLY, FULL COURSE)

_____

_____

OTHER DRUGS IN THIS CLASS

_____

_____

ADDITIONAL MEDICATIONS WITH SAME INDICATION

_____

_____

_____

ADVANTAGES/DISADVANTAGES COMPARED TO DRUGS LISTED ABOVE (CLASS, INDICATION)

_____

_____

_____

_____

CHAPTER 34

Ear Medications

LEARNING OBJECTIVES

After completing this chapter, you should be able to

1. Review the anatomy of the ear

2. Describe various ear disorders, including signs and symptoms, goals of treatment, and general treatment options

3. Identify medications used in the ear to treat cerumen buildup, water-clogged ears, contact dermatitis, and otitis media

4. List medications that can cause ototoxicity

5. Describe how to properly administer eardrops

PRONUNCIATIONS

Auditory (AW-di-tawr-ee)

Auricle (AWR-ih-kuhl)

Cerumen (sih-ROO-mun)

Equilibrium (ee-kwuh-LIB-ree-um)

Eustachian (yoo-STAY-shun)

Oscillopsia (os-ih-LOP-see-ah)

Otosclerosis (oh-tuh-skli-ROH-sis)

Ototoxicity (oh-toe-tok-SIS-eh-tee)

Tinnitus (TIN-ih-tus)

Tympanic (tim-PAN-ik)

Tympanostomy (tim-pan-OSS-toe-mee)

Matching

*Match each brand name ear drop with its primary ingredient(s) and regulatory status (**RX** or **OTC**). For additional study, list the indication for each product.*

Brands Names	Ingredients	Status	Indication
1. Auro-DRI			
2. Auroguard			
3. Cipro HC			
4. Coly-Mycin S			
5. Debrox			
6. Murine			
7. Otix			
8. Swim-EAR			

ACTIVE INGREDIENT(S)

a. Antipyrine/benzocaine

b. Carbamide peroxide

c. Hydrocortisone/ciprofloxacin

d. Hydrocortisone/neomycin/colistin

e. Isopropyl alcohol

True or False

For additional study, try to change the false statements to make them true.

_____1.   OTC carbamide peroxide eardrops are the safest way to treat children under the age of 6 for excess earwax.

_____2.   Swimmer's ear is an infection that may be treated with eardrops containing a combination of antibiotics and corticosteroids.

_____3.   Children with otitis media are usually treated with antibiotic eardrops.

_____4.   Ototoxicity from medications is the most common cause of hearing loss.

_____5.   Anesthetic eardrops may be a good treatment for painful ear infections without a fever.

Short Answer

1.   What are ear candles? Is the pharmacist likely to recommend them for patient use? Why or why not?

2.   What kinds of medications cause ototoxicity and hearing loss that may be permanent? Which drugs may cause temporary hearing loss?

3.   Describe the proper method for administration of otic (ear) drops.

CHAPTER 35

Mouth, Throat, and Nose Medications

LEARNING OBJECTIVES

After completing this chapter, you should be able to

1. Review the physiology of the upper respiratory system

2. Describe mouth irritations and treatments commonly used

3. Describe various upper respiratory tract disorders, including differentiating symptoms, duration of symptoms, and general treatment options

4. Identify medications used for benefit in the nose, mouth, and throat along with their therapeutic effects, most common side effects and adverse reactions, and mechanisms of action

5. Discuss local treatment options for sore throat

6. Discuss local treatment options for allergies and colds

Matching I

Match the following mouth care brand name products to their active ingredients and indications. For additional study, list the action of each product.

Brand Names	Ingredients	Indications	Actions
1. Anbesol			
2. Cepastat			
3. Chloraseptic			
4. Gly-Oxide			
5. Orajel			
6. Peridex			
7. Periogard			
8. Peroxyl			
9. Xylocaine			

ACTIVE INGREDIENTS

a. Benzocaine

b. Carbamide peroxide

c. Chlorhexidine

d. Hydrogen peroxide

e. Phenol

f. Lidocaine

INDICATIONS

G = Gingivitis

I = Mouth irritation

P = Mouth pain or irritation

PRONUNCIATIONS

Anesthetic (ann-es-THEH-tik)

Antihistamine (ann-tih-HIST-a-meen)

Antitussive (an-tih-TUSS-iv)

Decongestant (dee-kon-JES-tunt)

Expectorant (eks-PEK-ter-unt)

Gingivitis (jin-jih-VIE-tus)

Immunoglobulin E (im-MYOO-noh-GLOB-yoo-lin)

Larynx (LAYR-inks)

Methemoglobinemia (met-HEE-muh-gloh-bin-EEM-ee-ah)

Pharyngitis (fayr-in-JIE-tis)

Pharynx (FAYR-inks)

Plaque (plak)

Rhinitis (rye-NYE-tis)

Rhinorrhea (rye-nor-EE-huh)

Rhinovirus (RYE-noh-vye-ris)

Troches (TROH-keez)

Vasoconstriction (VAY-zoh-kon-STRIK-shun)

Matching II

Match each congestion/allergy brand name product to its active ingredient and route of administration. For additional study, write the class/action of each medication.

Brand Names	Ingredients	Route	Class/Action
1. Afrin			
2. Allegra			
3. Astelin			
4. Astepro			
5. Benadryl			
6. Benzedrex			
7. Chlor-Trimeton			
8. Clarinex			
9. Claritin			
10. NasalCrom			
11. Neo-Synephrine			
12. Privine			
13. Sudafed			
14. Sudafed PE			
15. Tavist			
16. Tyzine			
17. Xyzal			
18. Zyrtec			

ACTIVE INGREDIENTS

a. Azelastine
b. Cetirizine
c. Chlorpheniramine
d. Clemastine
e. Cromolyn
f. Desloratadine
g. Diphenhydramine
h. Fexofenadine

i. Levocetirizine
j. Loratadine
k. Naphazoline
l. Oxymetazoline
m. Phenylephrine
n. Propylhexedrine
o. Pseudoephedrine
p. Tetrahydrozoline

ROUTE OF ADMINISTRATION

X = Nasal
Y = Oral

True or False

For additional study, try to change the false statements to make them true.

_____1. Canker sores and mouth ulcers can often be treated with OTC products recommended by the pharmacist.

_____2. Thrush is a fungal infection for which the pharmacist can usually recommend an OTC treatment.

_____3. Local anesthetics for mouth and throat pain are safe and effective and should be used as frequently and continued as long as necessary to provide relief for sore throat pain.

_____4. Rhinitis may be caused by infection or allergy, but the treatment is usually directed at the symptoms.

_____5. Rebound congestion refers to an increase in congestion occurring after a missed dose of decongestant nasal drops.

_____6. Corticosteroids for nasal allergies are available only by prescription.

_____7. Colds are viral infections but can be cured using antihistamines and nasal decongestants.

_____8. Nasal corticosteroids and mast cell stabilizers are usually not helpful in controlling cold symptoms.

_____9. Many antihistamines and decongestants are available without a prescription but should not be given to children under the age of 4.

_____10. OTC products for cough and cold symptoms can safely be used together with medications for pain relief, especially those obtained with a prescription.

Short Answer

1. What is the function of an expectorant? What must a patient do to maximize its effectiveness?

2. What recommendations might a pharmacist make for a patient with a dry, hacking cough? How do they differ from those for a patient with a moist "productive" cough?

3. What group of patients should take special precautions in choosing OTC cold products? What advice might the pharmacist give to help them?

4. Compare the advantages and disadvantages of oral decongestants and antihistamines with those of nasally administered products.

5. What limitations are involved in the sale of OTC decongestant products containing pseudoephedrine? Why are these necessary?

DRUG MONOGRAPH

*Choose one brand name nasal corticosteroid (from **Medication Table 35-3**) and complete a drug monograph using the form provided here. (An example of the drug monograph is included in Chapter 1 of this workbook.)*

Generic Name _____

Brand Name _____

Manufacturer _____

APPROVED INDICATION(S)

_____
_____
_____
_____

DOSAGE AND ROUTE(S) OF ADMINISTRATION

_____
_____
_____

AVAILABLE DOSAGE FORM(S) STRENGTH(S)

STORAGE/HANDLING CONDITIONS/PROCEDURES

_____
_____
_____

PRECAUTIONS (CONTRAINDICATIONS, DRUG/FOOD INTERACTIONS, PREGNANCY CATEGORY)

_____
_____
_____
_____
_____
_____

COMMON OR SEVERE ADVERSE REACTIONS

_____
_____
_____
_____
_____

INSTRUCTIONS FOR PATIENTS

_____
_____
_____
_____
_____

COST OF THERAPY (DAILY, MONTHLY, FULL COURSE)

_____
_____
_____

OTHER DRUGS IN THIS CLASS

_____
_____
_____
_____

ADDITIONAL MEDICATIONS WITH SAME INDICATION

_____
_____
_____
_____

ADVANTAGES/DISADVANTAGES COMPARED TO DRUGS LISTED ABOVE (CLASS, INDICATION)

_____
_____
_____
_____
_____

Answer Key

CHAPTER 1

Why Technicians Need to Study Pharmacology and Therapeutics

Matching

Terms	Definitions
c	Agent used in the diagnosis, treatment, or prevention of disease
b	State of equilibrium of the internal environment of the body that is maintained by dynamic processes of feedback and regulation
d	Study of drugs
e	Study of expected results, dosages, side effects, and toxicities of agents used in the diagnosis, treatment, or prevention of disease
f	Study of the harmful effects of substances on the human body
a	Substance that may be expected to change or influence processes occurring in a living organism

True or False

For additional study, try to change the false statements to make them true.

1. **F** The study of pharmacology can help students gain a full understanding of the body and its processes.

2. **T**

3. **F** Pharmacy technicians frequently apply knowledge of pharmacology to their work.

4. **T**

5. **T**

6. **F** Knowledge of pharmacology is important in promoting patient safety.

7. **F** Pharmacy technicians should be prepared to communicate with other healthcare providers, including nurses, physicians, and dieticians.

8. **F** Pharmacists who have the support of well-educated pharmacy technicians may have more time to use their own knowledge for better patient care.

9. **T**

10. **T**

Short Answer

1. The technician in the case study uses his or her knowledge of pharmacology throughout the prescription filling process. The technician may need to know the correct spelling of the drug prescribed or its generic version in order to enter it into the computer, and he or she must understand the correlation between the directions on the prescription and the dosage form provided to the patient. Knowing pharmacology, he or she can better assist the pharmacist in affixing appropriate warning labels to the dispensing container. The technician can also determine when it is appropriate to refer a patient to the pharmacist for additional counseling on the use of the medication if that requires information beyond what is conveyed on the dispensing label.

2. a. The *indication* is the reason the drug is prescribed. A *contraindication* is a patient condition that makes use of this drug more dangerous, signaling that the drug should be avoided. An *adverse reaction* is a problem that occurs as a result of using the medication.

    b. A drug/food interaction is an undesirable effect that can occur when certain foods are consumed by patients taking a particular medication.

    c. *Pregnancy Category* gives an indication of whether a medication has been studied for use in pregnant women and/or the effects it might have on the developing fetus.

CHAPTER 2

Pharmacokinetics

Matching I

Definitions	Terms
1. Change or breakdown of a drug by the body's enzymes	i
2. Drugs that have a large fraction of the active drug metabolized before reaching the systemic circulation	g
3. Elimination of the drug and/or its metabolites from the body	f
4. Fraction of the administered dose that is available to the systemic circulation	b
5. How much drug will be given how often	e
6. Method of giving a drug	l
7. Movement of a drug from systemic circulation to its points of concentration throughout the body	d
8. Movement of a drug from the point of administration into the systemic circulation	a
9. Point in therapy when the amount of drug administered exactly replaces the amount of drug removed	m
10. Range of drug concentrations for which the majority of patients show effective therapeutic response with minimal drug-related side effects	n
11. Study of the body's effect on a drug	j
12. Substance that must be converted into an active form by the body, usually by an enzyme	k
13. Time it takes for one half of the drug to be removed from the body	h
14. Volume of serum, plasma, or blood that has all of the drug removed per unit of time by the eliminating organ	c

Matching II

Route of Administration	Common Abbreviation
1. Inhalation	b
2. Intramuscular	a
3. Intravenous	c
4. Oral (by mouth)	d
5. Rectal	e
6. Sublingual	g
7. Vaginal	f

True or False

1. **F** Application of pharmacokinetics allows pharmacists and physicians to predict what effects a particular dose of a drug might have on a patient.

2. **T**

3. **F** When possible, medications are administered by the route the patient prefers, but some drugs have limitations and require administration by particular routes (such as injection or rectal) that the patient may not prefer.

4. **T**

5. **F** Medications administered under the tongue take a shorter time to produce an action than those that are swallowed.

6. **F** Topical application is the term used for medications administered for use directly on the skin, into the eye, into the ear, and into the nose.

7. **T**

8. **F** Transdermal administration works for many drugs used to treat systemic (body-wide) conditions.

9. **T**

10. **T**

Short Answer

1. Application of pharmacokinetics to patient drug regimens allows the pharmacist to monitor drug concentrations that correlate with drug effects, both therapeutic and toxic. These concentrations can be measured through blood draws. Calculations can be utilized to estimate concentrations at any time after a drug is given.

2. Metabolites are compounds formed as a result of the breakdown of drugs by the body's enzyme systems. Metabolites may be active or inactive when compared to their precursors and may even be responsible for toxic side effects. Some drugs are inactive until they are activated by being metabolized.

Drug Monograph

1. Atorvastatin is administered orally, meaning it is taken by mouth.

2. Atorvastatin must be absorbed from the gastrointestinal tract into the bloodstream, where it reduces the risk of heart attack and stroke by lowering a patient's cholesterol.

3. Consumption of high fiber foods with atorvastatin may lower the amount that is absorbed from the GI tract into the bloodstream, decreasing its effectiveness in lowering cholesterol.

CHAPTER 3

The Autonomic Nervous System

Matching I

SANS	Bladder sphincter contraction	SANS	Decreased gland secretion
PANS	Bladder sphincter relaxation	SANS	Decreased gastro-intestinal motility
SANS	Blood vessel constriction	PANS	Decreased heart rate
PANS	Blood vessel dilation	SANS	Dilation of pupils (mydriasis)
PANS	Bronchoconstriction	PANS	Increased gastro-intestinal motility
SANS	Bronchodilation	PANS	Increased gland secretion
PANS	Constriction of pupils (miosis)	SANS	Increased heart rate

Matching II

Brand Names	Generic Names	Indications
1. Atrovent	h	COPD
2. Bentyl	d	bowel disorders
3. Cogentin	b	Parkinson's symptoms
4. Detrol	l	overactive bladder
5. Ditropan XL	i	neurogenic bladder
6. Donnatal	a	irritable bowel syndrome
7. Enablex	c	overactive bladder
8. Levsinex	g	bowel, bladder disorders
9. Robinul	f	control of airway secretions
10. Toviaz	e	overactive bladder
11. Transderm Scōp	j	motion sickness
12. VESIcare	k	overactive bladder

True or False

For additional study, try to change the false statements to make them true.

1. **T**

2. **F** The SANS is often called the adrenergic nervous system.

3. **F** There are three main types of adrenergic receptors, α_1, β_1, and β_2.

4. **T**

5. **F** Epinephrine is a natural (endogenous) neurotransmitter that stimulates adrenergic receptors.

6. **T**

7. **T**

8. **F** β_1 antagonists interfere most with the actions of the SANS on the heart and blood vessels.

Short Answer

1. In many parts of the body (blood vessels, heart, lungs, eyes), the SANS and PANS have opposite actions. Anticholinergic medications oppose the actions of the PANS so their effects may resemble those of adrenergic medications that stimulate the SANS. For example, the SANS promotes bronchodilation, while PANS stimulation causes bronchoconstriction. An anticholinergic medication such as ipratropium blocks PANS-mediated bronchoconstriction, causing bronchodilation, the same effect which would be expected from a SANS agonist.

2. Pseudoephedrine is a medication that acts directly on adrenergic receptors and induces the release of NE, which also stimulates adrenergic receptors; adrenergic (SANS) stimulation causes constriction of vessels in the nasal passages, thus, relieving congestion. But it can also cause constriction of other blood vessels (all enervated by the SANS), which could increase blood pressure as well.

3. The main neurotransmitters of the SANS are norepinephrine and epinephrine, also known as *noradrenaline* and *adrenaline*. The term *adrenergic* comes from the alternate name for these neurotransmitters that are active in the SANS.

4. Although a nonspecific β antagonist will interfere with actions of the SANS on the heart and blood vessels that contribute to hypertension, it also interferes with SANS actions in the lungs (bronchodilation) and can contribute to asthma symptoms by causing bronchoconstriction. A selective β_1 blocker has less effect on the lungs and bronchi, where the SANS receptors are primarily of the β_2 type, and more effect on the heart and blood vessels, where the β_1 receptors are located.

5. The PANS promotes bladder sphincter relaxation. Too much PANS stimulation can relax it so much that the bladder becomes "overactive" and urination cannot be controlled. Antimuscarinic drugs work against PANS stimulation, allowing patients more control over the bladder sphincter.

CHAPTER 4

The Central Nervous System

Matching I

Neurotransmitters	Functions in CNS	Abbreviations
1. Acetylcholine	a	ACH
2. Dopamine	b	
3. Epinephrine	c	Epi
4. Gamma-amino butyric acid	f	GABA
5. Glutamate	g	
6. Histamine	d	H
7. Norepinephrine	c	NE
8. Serotonin	e	5-HT

Matching II

Brand Names	Generic Names	Analgesic/Anesthetic
1. Actiq	b	analgesic
2. Avinza	g	analgesic
3. Demerol	f	analgesic
4. Dilaudid	c	analgesic
5. Diprivan	j	anesthetic
6. Duragesic	b	analgesic
7. Kadian	g	analgesic
8. Ketalar	d	anesthetic
9. Lidoderm	e	anesthetic
10. Marcaine	a	anesthetic
11. MS Contin	g	analgesic
12. Novocain	i	anesthetic
13. OxyContin	h	analgesic
14. Pontocaine	k	anesthetic
15. Roxanol	g	analgesic
16. Sensorcaine	a	anesthetic
17. Sublimaze	b	analgesic
18. Ultram	l	analgesic

True or False

For additional study, try to change the false statements to make them true.

1. **F** The CNS includes the brain and spinal cord. The SANS and PANS are parts of the autonomic nervous system.

2. **T**

3. **T**

4. **F** Local anesthetics are applied to a specific part of the body to block the nerves in that part of the body.

5. **F** Propofol injections are white and opaque in appearance, similar to milk because they consist of a fat emulsion.

6. **T**

7. **F** Opioid analgesics are often combined with a non-opioid such as acetaminophen or an NSAID to increase pain relieving potency.

8. **T**

9. **T**

10. **F** Naltrexone is a long-acting opiate antagonist used in the management of addiction.

Short Answer

1. The BBB is formed by a row of specialized cells in the blood vessels that feed the brain and help produce CSF. It keeps foreign organisms and chemicals from entering the brain while still allowing nutrients and oxygen to enter. Medications that have actions in the CNS generally need to cross the BBB to cause their action.

2. The cell body of a neuron is called the soma. This is where proteins and neurotransmitters are made and where the nucleus resides. Branching directly off of the soma are structures called dendrites. Dendrites receive information from other cells as transmitted by action potentials and the release of neurotransmitters. Axons are the part of the nerve that stretches away from the body of the nerve cell to carry signals to the next nerve and are sometimes coated in a myelin sheath or a layer of fat and protein that protects the axon and increases the conduction of nerve impulses. The point at which the axon ends is a space called the synapse where neurotransmitters are released in order for the action potential to send information to other neurons.

3. Epidural anesthesia is when a local anesthetic is injected into the epidural space in the spinal cord to block the spinal nerve roots thus causing decreased sensation.

   One advantage to using epidural anesthesia is the ability to place a catheter into the epidural space to administer a continuous dose of local anesthetic. This eliminates the need to give repeated injections into the epidural space. In patients who have pain, opioids can be administered with the local anesthetic into the epidural space to give even longer lasting pain relief. Even in patients who are postoperative, the combination of an opioid and local anesthetic administered in the epidural space may be enough to provide adequate pain relief.

4. Tolerance is defined as needing larger doses of medication for the same effect. This does not necessarily result in addiction. Physical dependence is defined as the occurrence of withdrawal symptoms upon abrupt reduction or discontinuation of the drug. (Withdrawal symptoms may also result with the administration of an antagonist medication.) Both tolerance and physical dependence are common occurrences in chronic users of opiate agonists and are very different from addiction. Addiction, also known as psychological dependence, is a behavioral pattern characterized by a lack of control over and compulsive use of drugs despite negative consequences.

5. PCA (patient-controlled analgesia) is a popular method of managing pain in the hospital setting. It allows the patient to self-administer opiate analgesia using preset parameters for dose and frequency. PCA is accomplished using an electronic intravenous pump attached to a button that the patient presses for pain control. Only a prespecified amount of medication is administered with each button press, and the patient is only allowed to press the button a certain number of times per hour. A PCA pump also includes a continuous infusion of a basal dose of analgesic. This method of administration results in better pain control and the patient feeling empowered.

CHAPTER 5

Neurologic Disorders

Matching I

Disorders	Associated Symptoms
1. Cluster headache	m, q
2. Dementia	b, e
3. Epilepsy	d, i
4. Migraine	j, r
5. Multiple sclerosis	f, h
6. Neuropathic pain	g, k
7. Parkinson's disease	a, s
8. Restless leg syndrome	c, p
9. Sleep apnea	f, l
10. Stroke	n, o

Matching II

Brand Names	Generic Names	Indications
1. Ambien	t	insomnia
2. Aricept	e	dementia
3. Artane	s	PD
4. Avonex	i	MS
5. Azilect	n	PD
6. Betaseron	j	MS
7. Cerebyx	g	seizures
8. Cogentin	a	PD
9. Cognex	p	dementia
10. Comtan	f	PD
11. Copaxone	h	MS
12. Depakote	d	seizures
13. Dilantin	m	seizures
14. Dostinex	b	PD
15. Exelon	o	dementia
16. Gabitril	q	seizures
17. Halcion	r	insomnia
18. Keppra	l	seizures
19. Klonopin	c	seizures
20. Lamictal	k	seizures

Matching III

Brand Names	Generic Names	Indications
1. Lunesta	d	insomnia
2. Lyrica	l	seizures, neuropathic pain
3. Mirapex	k	PD, RLS
4. Mysoline	m	seizures
5. Namenda	h	dementia
6. Neurontin	e	seizures, neuropathic pain
7. Parlodel	b	PD
8. Razadyne	f	dementia
9. Requip	o	PD, RLS
10. Restoril	p	insomnia
11. Rozerem	n	insomnia
12. Sinemet	c	PD
13. Sonata	s	insomnia
14. Symmetrel	a	PD
15. Tasmar	q	PD
16. Topamax	r	seizures
17. Trileptal	j	seizures
18. Tysabri	i	MS
19. Vimpat	g	seizures
20. Zonegran	t	seizures

True or False

1. **F** OTC pain medications can cause chronic daily headache if overused.

2. **T**

3. **F** A stroke caused by bleeding in the brain is known as hemorrhagic stroke.

4. **T**

5. **F** Dementia cannot be cured, although medications may help to slow its progress.

6. **F** The EEG is the most beneficial tool for detecting the abnormalities associated with epilepsy, but treatment is primarily medication.

7. **F** Pregabalin and gabapentin are useful in the treatment of seizures AND for neuropathic pain.

8. **T**

Short Answer

1. The approach to managing migraine headaches is both to try to prevent them (prophylactic therapy) and to treat the headache when it occurs. Treating the headache at the first sign of onset is usually more effective at getting rid of it than waiting to try to treat a full-blown migraine. Prophylactic medications include beta blockers (atenolol, propranolol, metoprolol), tricyclic antidepressants (desipramine, nortriptyline, and amitriptyline), and antiepileptic drugs (valproate and topiramate) and are used to prevent migraines.

   Usually drugs used for prevention must be taken for several weeks to get the best effects.

   Patients need to be patient and keep a headache diary to monitor benefits.

2. For patients who have not had recent surgery or bleeding problems, a thrombotic stroke that has occurred less than 3 hours ago can be treated with alteplase (tPA or tissue plasminogen activator) to break up the clot that has caused a stroke. Alteplase is administered by IV infusion as soon as the patient has been deemed to qualify for its use. Because alteplase can dissolve any clots in the body, a patient who has had recent surgery or bleeding problems usually cannot take this drug. Stroke patients are also routinely started on antiplatelet therapy to reduce the risk of another clot forming. Antiplatelet agents used include aspirin, clopidogrel, and dipyridamole. In addition, stroke patients are usually started on a statin drug, which has been shown to reduce the occurrence of future strokes.

3. All drugs that increase dopamine activity, including both dopamine agonists and levodopa, have the potential to cause hallucinations, dyskinesias (abnormal movements), and unusual obsessive behavior. Some patients taking these medicines have developed a new compulsion to gamble or obsession with sex. In addition, these medicines have a blackbox warning regarding "sleep attacks." There are reports of patients suddenly, without preliminary drowsiness, falling asleep. Patients should be warned of this possibility, especially if they are still operating automobiles or machinery. Tolcapone has reports of liver damage.

4. Vitamin E and the herb gingko biloba have been studied to see if they would benefit patients with Alzheimer's disease. Vitamin E was hypothesized to work as an antioxidant to reduce the advancement of the disease. Gingko biloba, a plant used for centuries in traditional Chinese medicine, was thought to be beneficial by acting to enhance neurotransmitter activity, improve blood circulation in the brain, or other unknown actions.

   Studies have not shown a clear benefit for either, but some doctors will use high doses of vitamin E. When gingko biloba is used, it should be used early in the course of the disease. Although not standard medications, both vitamin E and gingko biloba still have the potential for side effects and drug interactions.

5. Good sleep hygiene refers to nonpharmacologic measures that improve the ability to fall and stay asleep. These include a regular sleep schedule, avoidance of evening alcohol and long naps, using the bed only for sleep and intimacy, and regular exercise.

Matching I

Disorders	Associated Symptoms
1. Anxiety disorders	**f, h**
2. ADHD	**a, b**
3. Bipolar disorder	**c, d, e**
4. Depression	**i, j**
5. Schizophrenia	**c, g**

Matching II

Brand Names	Generic Names	Indications	Medication Class
1. Adderall	**j**	**A**	stimulant
2. Celexa	**c**	**D**	SSRI
3. Concerta	**i**	**A**	stimulant
4. Daytrana	**i**	**A**	stimulant
5. Effexor	**l**	**D**	SNRI
6. Elavil	**a**	**D**	tricyclic
7. Intuniv	**g**	**A**	nonstimulant
8. Lexapro	**e**	**D**	SSRI
9. Pristiq	**d**	**D**	SNRI
10. Prozac	**f**	**D**	SSRI
11. Ritalin	**i**	**A**	stimulant
12. Strattera	**b**	**A**	nonstimulant
13. Vyvanse	**h**	**A**	stimulant
14. Zoloft	**k**	**D**	SSRI

Matching III

Brand Names	Generic Names	Indications
1. Abilify	**c**	antipsychotic
2. Antabuse	**h**	substance abuse
3. Ativan	**k**	anxiety
4. Campral	**a**	substance abuse
5. Chantix	**o**	smoking cessation
6. Clozaril	**f**	antipsychotic

7. Haldol	**j**	antipsychotic
8. Nicoderm	**l**	smoking cessation
9. Nicorette	**l**	smoking cessation
10. Prolixin	**i**	antipsychotic
11. Risperdal	**n**	antipsychotic
12. Suboxone	**d**	substance abuse
13. Valium	**g**	anxiety, seizures
14. Xanax	**b**	anxiety
15. Zyban	**e**	smoking cessation
16. Zyprexa	**m**	antipsychotic

True or False

1. **F** Psychiatric disorders, for the most part, cannot be detected using blood tests or standard diagnostic procedures but are expressed in terms of emotions and behaviors.

2. **T**

3. **T**

4. **F** Patients who take benzodiazepines need to be warned that these medications can reduce alertness and make driving or operating machinery hazardous.

5. **F** Schizophrenia is a disease that is lifelong and has no cure, but medication therapy can control and reduce symptoms

6. **T**

7. **T**

8. **F** Lithium is the oldest and best studied medication for bipolar disorder

9. **F** About 2/3 of children with ADHD will continue to have symptoms into adulthood.

10. **F** Addiction is a chronic, compulsive craving for a drug, while dependence means a patient may have withdrawal symptoms once the drug is stopped. Patients can be addicted without dependence and dependent without being addicted.

Short Answer

1. Psychiatric disorders, for the most part, cannot be detected or monitored using blood tests, X-rays, or any number of diagnostic procedures in the way other medical problems are. Symptoms of these disorders are expressed in terms of emotions and behaviors. People with neurologic diseases and those with psychiatric diagnoses are burdened with stigma—the condition of associating negative attitudes with a person due to a characteristic that person carries. The stigma of psychiatric disorders can cause delays in diagnosis and adherence to treatment. Psychiatric patients are sometimes blamed for their conditions, believed to be morally lacking, and told that they are weak. Patients are subjected to scrutiny and judgment that those with other medical conditions, such as diabetes and cancer, do not have to deal with.

2. The main classes of antidepressants are selective serotonin reuptake inhibitors (SSRIs, which include sertraline, paroxetine, and citalopram), serotonin norepinephrine reuptake inhibitors (SNRIs, which include desvenlafaxine, venlafaxine, and duloxetine), monoamine oxidase inhibitors (MAOIs, including phenelzine, pargyline, and tranylcypromine), and tricyclic antidepressants (TCAs, including amitriptyline, desipramine, and doxepin). All increase neurotransmitter levels (although in different ways) and are delayed in acting, so they must be taken for a few weeks before their full effect is seen.

3. Benzodiazepines used to treat anxiety include shorter-acting drugs like alprazolam and lorazepam and longer-acting ones like diazepam and clonazepam. Triazepam, temazepam, and flurazepam are specifically indicated for insomnia.

4. Typical antipsychotics include chlorpromazine, thioridazine, haloperidol, and fluphenazine. They have anticholinergic side effects (dry mouth, constipation, urinary retention) and extrapyramidal (Parkinson-like) side effects. Atypical antipsychotics include risperidone, olanzapine, quetiapine, aripiprazole, and ziprasidone, which have side effects like weight gain, glucose intolerance, and lipid abnormalities.

5. Lithium is a mood stabilizer used primarily to treat bipolar disorders. Other mood stabilizers include valproate, lamotrigine, and carbamazepine, also used for the treatment of epilepsy.

CHAPTER 7

Overview of the Endocrine System and Agents

Matching I

Disorders	Symptoms	Treatments
Acromegaly	a	2
Hyperparathyroidism	b	4
Hyperthyroidism	d	3
Hypothyroidism	c	1

Matching II

Brand Names	Generic Names	Conditions
1. Forteo	h	osteoporosis
2. Levoxyl	e	hypothyroidism
3. Miacalcin	b	osteoporosis
4. Parlodel	a	acromegaly
5. PhosLo	d	secondary hyperparathyroidism
6. Renagel	g	SHPT
7. Rocaltrol	c	HP, PHP, SHPT
8. Sandostatin	f	acromegaly
9. Synthroid	e	hypothyroidism

True or False

1. **F** One function of hormones in the body is to regulate sexual characteristics, but hormones are released from many different glands and are active in many bodily functions and actions.

2. **F** The thyroid gland has two lobes and is located in the anterior of the neck. OR The pituitary gland has two lobes and is located in the brain.

3. **T**

4. **T**

5. **F** A condition caused by excess growth hormone (GH) production is acromegaly.

6. **F** Octreotide is available as an intramuscular depot suspension injected every 5 weeks to control GH levels.

7. **F** Hyperthyroidism is treated with antithyroid preparations like methimazole or propylthiouracil.

8. **T**

9. **F** Calcitriol is a vitamin D metabolite used in treatment of patients deficient in PTH.

10. **T**

Short Answer

1. Anterior pituitary hormones include the trophic hormones LH and FSH that control production of the sex hormones, ACTH that acts on the adrenal gland, and TSH that stimulates the production of thyroid hormones; nontrophic anterior pituitary hormones are GH, which induces growth in children, and prolactin, which stimulates milk production in lactating women. Posterior pituitary hormones are vasopressin, which is active in blood pressure control, and oxytocin, which induces uterine contractions and milk letdown.

2. The thyroid gland uses iodine to make the thyroid hormones T3 and T4 that work in every organ system to regulate the body's metabolism, affecting consumption of oxygen, production of heat, cardiac function, and growth and development.

3. The parathyroid produces PTH, which regulates calcium concentrations in the blood.

4. Patients with chronic kidney disease usually receive a combination of phosphate binders (such as sevelamer), calcium supplements (including calcium carbonate), vitamin D, and calcimimetics. These are prescribed to manage PTH, phosphate, and calcium balance to slow or prevent SHPT, renal osteodystrophy, and tissue calcification.

5. Vitamin D preparations include calcitriol, dihydrotachysterol, doxercalciferol, ergocalciferol, and paricalcitol. All are available in oral dosage forms. Some are also administered IV or IM.

CHAPTER 8

Adrenal Gland Hormones

Matching I

Actions	Hormones	Exogenous Hormone Medication
Anti-inflammatory effect	c	methylprednisolone, triamcinolone, dexamethasone
Immune response suppression	c	methylprednisolone, triamcinolone, dexamethasone
Potassium depletion	a	cortisone, hydrocortisone
Regulation of blood glucose	c	methylprednisolone, triamcinolone, dexamethasone
Sexual maturation	b	testosterone, fluoxymesterone
Sodium retention	a	cortisone, hydrocortisone
Water retention	a	cortisone, hydrocortisone

Matching II

Brand Names	Generic Names	Routes of Administration
1. Cortaid	d	topical
2. Cortef	d	oral
3. Cortifoam	d	rectal
4. Depo-Medrol	e	injection
5. Diprolene	a	topical
6. Elocon	f	topical
7. Kenalog	g	injection, topical
8. Medrol	e	oral
9. Solu-Cortef	d	injection
10. Solu-Medrol	e	injection
11. Synalar	c	topical
12. Topicort	b	topical

True or False

1. **T**

2. **F** ACTH secreted by the pituitary gland stimulates the adrenal glands.

3. **F** Cortisol is the primary glucocorticoid secreted by the adrenal glands

4. **T**

5. **F** The glucocorticoid medications are called steroids but are not the same as the anabolic steroids abused to build muscle mass and athletic performance.

6. **T**

7. **F** Allergic reactions are common indications for treatment with dermatologic corticosteroids.

8. **T**

9. **F** Hydrocortisone topical preparations are available over-the-counter.

10. **T**

Short Answer

1. The adrenal glands are small triangular-shaped organs located on top of both kidneys. Each consists of two main regions: the adrenal cortex, which makes up the outer region of the adrenal gland, and the adrenal medulla, which makes up the inner region of the adrenal gland. The inner medulla is responsible for secreting the hormones epinephrine and norepinephrine (also known as adrenaline and noradrenaline, respectively).

2. Exogenous glucocorticoid medications can be prescribed for a multitude of indications such as adrenal insufficiency, inflammatory conditions (e.g., some skin conditions, asthma, allergic rhinitis), and autoimmune diseases (e.g., rheumatoid arthritis).

3. (See **Medication Table 8-1**.) Methylprednisolone, triamcinolone, betamethasone, and dexamethasone have little or no mineralocorticoid activity. This means that they can be expected to cause less sodium and water retention than preparations (such as cortisone, hydrocortisone, and prednisone).

4. Cushing's Syndrome (hypercortisolism) is the disease that results from excessive amounts of glucocorticoids circulating in the body. It is usually treated with surgery or radiation, but some medications that inhibit steroidogenesis (corticosteroid production) may also be used. These include metyrapone, ketoconazole, etomidate, and mitotane.

5. Supplemental corticosteroids for acute adrenal insufficiency should be tapered gradually rather than abruptly discontinued.

CHAPTER 9

Diabetes

Matching I

Brand Names	Generic Names	Duration of Action
1. Apidra	d	R
2. Humalog	e	R
3. Humulin N	f	I
4. Humulin R	g	S
5. Lantus	c	L
6. Levemir	b	L
7. Novolin N	f	I
8. Novolin R	g	S
9. Novolog	a	R

Matching II

Brand Names	Generic Names	Routes	Mechanism of Action
1. Actos	f	Oral	Increases insulin sensitivity
2. Avandia	i	Oral	Increases insulin sensitivity
3. Byetta	a	Subcu-taneous	Increases insulin secretion/reduces glucose production
4. Gluco-phage	d	Oral	Increases insulin sensitivity
5. Glucotrol	b	Oral	Stimulates insulin production
6. Januvia	j	Oral	Increases insulin production
7. Prandin	h	Oral	Stimulates insulin production
8. Starlix	e	Oral	Stimulates insulin production
9. Symlin	g	Subcu-taneous	Inhibits glucagon release
10. Tradjenta	c	Oral	Increases insulin production

True or False

1. **F** Some Type 2 diabetes is related to a reduced sensitivity of the body's cells to the actions of insulin, but all Type 1 and some Type 2 diabetes are caused by a deficiency of insulin production.

2. **F** Complications of diabetes (including heart disease and stroke) may be life-threatening.

3. **T**

4. **F** Insulin injection sites should be rotated to prevent lipodystrophy and promote consistent absorption.

5. **T**

6. **F** Alpha-glucosidase inhibitors such as acarbose should be taken with meals, preferably along with the first bite of food.

7. **T**

8. **F** Metformin does not act on the beta cells in the pancreas or increase insulin production; it increases insulin sensitivity of cells in body tissues.

9. **F** Rosiglitazone has been associated with an increased risk of myocardial infarction and cardiac death. Sitagliptin has been associated with severe pancreatitis.

10. **F** Besides insulin, other diabetes therapies that are administered by injection include pramlintide, exenatide, and liraglutide.

Short Answer

1. Metabolic syndrome is a group of disorders characterized primarily by abdominal obesity accompanied by dyslipidemia, hypertension, and hyperglycemia. Patients with this disorder are at high risk for cardiovascular events such as myocardial infarction and stroke.

2. Insulin is necessary for every patient's metabolism. In Type 1 diabetes, the pancreatic cells that produce insulin have been destroyed and no longer produce this important hormone, so it must be supplied by injection in order for them to stay alive. Patients with Type 2 diabetes may still have some insulin production, just not enough for their metabolic needs, and can be treated with medications that either stimulate higher insulin production or reduce those metabolic needs.

3. Because insulin is a protein that would be digested (and thus inactivated) in the gastrointestinal tract, it cannot be administered by the oral route. Currently all available insulin products are given by injection.

4. SMBG is self-monitoring of blood glucose—testing small samples of blood to measure glucose levels. It can be used to track the success of a diabetes treatment regimen or even to make adjustments in medication doses for better glycemic control or side effect (hypoglycemia) management.

5. Hypoglycemia is the most common side effect of diabetes medications other than the alpha glucosidase inhibitors (pramlintide and exenatide). This is not surprising because these medications are intended to lower blood glucose.

CHAPTER 10

Reproductive Hormones

Matching I

Hormones	Functions	Gland/ Organ	Full Name
1. Estrogen	b	O	
2. FSH	d	P	follicle-stimulating hormone
3. GnRH	f	H	gonadotropin-releasing hormone
4. LH	e	P	luteinizing hormone
5. Progesterone	a	O	
6. Testosterone	c	T	

Matching II

Brand Names	Generic Names	Indications
1. Androderm	o	male hormone replacement
2. AndroGel	o	male hormone replacement
3. Angeliq	i	female hormone replacement
4. Avodart	d	BPH
5. Casodex	a	prostate cancer
6. Depo-Provera	m	contraception
7. Flomax	n	BPH
8. Gianvi	f	contraception
9. Loestrin 24 FE	g	contraception
10. Lupron	l	prostate cancer
11. NuvaRing	e	contraception
12. Ocella	f	contraception
13. Premarin	b	female hormone replacement
14. Prempro	c	female hormone replacement
15. Proscar	k	BPH
16. Provera	m	female hormone replacement
17. TriNessa-28	h	contraception

18. Tri-Sprintec	h	contraception
19. Vivelle	j	female hormone replacement
20. Yaz	f	contraception

True or False

1. **F** Menopause is the time of a woman's life when menstruation and ovulation cease.

2. **T**

3. **T**

4. **F** A four-phasic contraceptive regimen is one with four different dose combinations of estrogen and progesterone over a 29-day cycle.

    OR: An extended cycle regimen may reduce the frequency of menses to four times per year.

5. **F** Hormonal contraceptives can be inserted vaginally (NuvaRing), administered transdermally (Ortho Evra), or injected (Depo-Provera), as well as being taken by mouth.

6. **F** Emergency contraception must be started within 72 hours of unprotected intercourse. Some preparations, including Plan B, are available OTC.

7. **T**

8. **T**

9. **F** Transdermal and intravaginal estrogen treatment is less likely to result in side effects than oral therapy because less estrogen reaches systemic circulation.

10. **T**

Short Answer

1. Common side effects associated with COCs are related to the dose of estrogen as well as the activity of the progestin. Estrogenic effects include nausea, breast tenderness, increased blood pressure, and headache. Progestogenic effects include breast tenderness, headache, fatigue, and mood changes. Androgenic effects include increased appetite, weight gain, acne, oily skin, hirsutism, and cholesterol abnormalities. In addition to these common side effects, patients should be counseled regarding the possibility for more serious adverse effects. Although not common in younger women, estrogen and progestin can increase a woman's risk for blood clots, heart attacks, and strokes.

2. FDA requires a medication guide with information regarding proper use of the medications, common and serious side effects, management of side effects, and when to seek medical attention. Additionally, women should receive information reminding them that contraceptives do not protect against STDs.

3. The Yuzpe method is a combined oral contraceptive regimen, which uses 100 mcg of ethinyl estradiol and 0.5 mg of levonorgestrel per dose administered as two doses 12 hours apart. Similarly, Trivora® may be used for EC by taking 4 pink tablets followed by 4 pink tablets 12 hours later. The Yuzpe method is approximately 75% effective in reducing the incidence of unplanned pregnancies. The most common adverse effect associated with the Yuzpe method is nausea. Many patients are counseled to take an antiemetic one hour before the EC dose is taken.

4. Clomiphene citrate is indicated for the treatment of infertility and works by stimulating ovulation. The most common side effects are ovarian enlargement, flushing, abdominal discomfort, bloating, nausea, vomiting, breast discomfort, and visual disturbances. Its most dangerous side effect is ovarian hyperstimulation syndrome.

5. BPH stands for benign prostatic hyperplasia, a non-cancerous enlargement of the prostate gland affecting mostly elderly males. The most common symptoms are urinary tract disturbances, and it is treated with alpha-1 receptor blockers such as tamsulosin or 5-alpha reductase inhibitors such as finasteride.

CHAPTER 11

Overview of the Musculoskeletal System

Matching I

Brand Names	Generic Names	Class (S or N)	Injectable Available?
1. Anectine	l	N	inj
2. Dantrium	g	S	inj
3. Flexeril	f	S	
4. Lioresal	a	S	inj
5. Nimbex	e	N	inj
6. Norflex	j	S	inj
7. Parafon Forte	d	S	
8. Quelicin	l	N	inj
9. Robaxin	i	S	inj
10. Skelaxin	h	S	
11. Soma Compound	c	S	
12. Soma	b	S	
13. Zanaflex	m	S	
14. Zemuron	k	N	inj

Matching II

Medications	Side/Adverse Effects
1. atracurium	c
2. chlorzoxazone	f
3. cisatracurium	a
4. cyclobenzaprine	b
5. methocarbamol	f
6. orphenadrine	b
7. succinylcholine	e
8. tizanidine	d

True or False

1. **F** Musculoskeletal pain is one of the most common medical complaints among adult patients.

2. **T**

3. **F** The first-line treatment for muscle strain is acetaminophen or a NSAID.

4. **F** Antispasmodic agents are usually prescribed to treat chronic conditions causing generalized muscle cramping, increased muscle tone, or spasticity.

5. **T**

6. **F** Bed rest is not recommended for treatment of acute low back pain related to a muscle strain.

7. **F** Intravenous dantrolene must be reconstituted immediately before use.

8. **T**

9. **F** Succinylcholine is an ultra-short-acting neuromuscular blocking agent.

10. **F** Nondepolarizing neuromuscular blockers are associated with serious adverse effects including anaphylaxis, bronchiole constriction, and decreases in blood pressure.

Short Answer

1. A sprain is an abnormal stretching or tear of a ligament that can result in swelling, pain, and even bruising. A common example is a twisted ankle that can result in the sprain of the ligament(s) and may cause pain and swelling of the area on the outside of the ankle. Sometimes, it can even cause some bruising, which is evidence of very small tears in the ligament(s) that is overstretched. A strain is an overstretched muscle or tendon that is often twisted, pulled, or even slightly torn. Overuse of a muscle or repetitive use can also cause a muscle strain. Muscle strains can result in pain of the injured muscle as well as the surrounding muscles. It may also cause swelling, cramping, or even muscle spasm.

2. A muscle spasm can occur as a result of strain and contribute to the pain a patient feels. Spasmolytics decrease the spasm and break the pain-spasm cycle sometimes found in back pain due to strain.

3. Most commonly centrally-acting spasmolytics may cause dizziness, drowsiness, lightheadedness, fatigue, dry mouth, or nausea. For this reasons patients should not drive or operate heavy machinery while using these medications. There is also a potential for abuse and/or dependency, so patients should be reminded to take them only as directed.

4. Chronic conditions like cerebral palsy, multiple sclerosis, spinal cord injury, and stroke damage can cause increased muscle tone or spasticity that may be relieved to some extent by antispasmodic medications.

5. In the emergency room or operating room, when an endotracheal tube is placed, it is better to have a paralyzing agent that will wear off quickly and have less potential for side effects. If longer periods of paralysis are required during longer surgeries or when sedation is needed, a longer-acting agent may have better effects and require less frequent dosing.

CHAPTER 12

Musculoskeletal Disorders

Matching I

Conditions	Symp-toms	Cause
1. Gouty arthritis	b	high uric acid levels/uric acid crystals
2. Osteoarthritis	d	degraded joint cartilage
3. Osteoporosis	a	low bone density
4. Rheumatoid arthritis	e	autoimmune inflammation
5. Systemic lupus erythematosus	c	autoimmune inflammation

Matching II

Brand Names	Generic Names	Indica-tion	Route of Administration
1. Actonel	m	O	PO
2. Boniva	i	O	PO, IV
3. Colcrys	e	T	PO
4. Enbrel	f	R	SQ
5. Forteo	n	O	SQ
6. Fortical	d	O	Nasal
7. Fosamax	b	O	PO
8. Humira	a	R	SQ
9. Krystexxa	l	T	IV
10. Miacalcin	d	O	IM, nasal
11. Plaquenil	h	R	PO
12. Remicade	j	R	SQ
13. Rheumatrex	k	R	PO, SQ, IV
14. Uloric	g	T	PO
15. Zyloprim	c	T	PO, IV

Matching III

Brand Names	Generic Names	NSAIDs
1. Advil	e	NSAID
2. Aleve	f	NSAID
3. Celebrex	b	NSAID
4. Dolobid	d	NSAID
5. Flector	c	NSAID
6. Motrin	e	NSAID
7. Rybix	g	
8. Tylenol	a	
9. Ultram	g	
10. Voltaren	c	NSAID

True or False

1. **T**

2. **F** High uric acid levels do not always lead to gout attacks, so patients should only be treated with medication during an attack or to prevent future attacks.

3. **F** Pegloticase may be administered only in a health-care setting where professionals are prepared to deal with potentially life-threatening adverse reactions.

4. **T**

5. **F** Oral bisphosphonates are not absorbed very well. Patients should take them first thing in the morning on an empty stomach with a large glass of water. After taking the tablet, they should refrain from eating and remain upright for an additional 30 minutes.

6. **T**

7. **F** Rheumatoid arthritis is treated with corticosteroids, NSAIDs, and DMARDs.

8. **T**

9. **F** Biologic DMARDs carry a black box warning about the risk of tuberculosis and invasive fungal infections.

10. **T**

Short Answer

1. Most of the medications used to prevent gout attacks lower uric acid levels, either by increasing excretion (like probenecid) or decreasing production (like allopurinol and febuxostat). Pegloticase reduces uric acid levels by converting uric acid to allantoin, which is then excreted.

2. Vitamin D is necessary for calcium to be absorbed and used by the body. Although it is produced naturally when people are exposed to sunlight and is also added to fortified dairy products, some patients still do not get enough, especially during winter months or when dairy intake is limited.

3. Glucosamine and chondroitin are over-the-counter nutritional supplements found to be beneficial for some patients with moderate to severe pain from OA. The usual dose is a total of 1500 mg glucosamine and 1200 mg chondroitin daily. They are not part of standard therapy because the mechanism of action is unclear and there is mixed evidence regarding effectiveness.

4. DMARD stands for Disease-Modifying Anti-Rheumatic Drug. All work by decreasing different inflammatory mediators within the body to reduce RA disease activity.

5. SLE can affect the joints, skin, CNS, lungs, heart, kidneys, and hematologic systems, all as a result of the immune system attacking body tissues.

CHAPTER 13

Overview of the Cardiovascular and Renal Systems

Matching I

Label	#	Function
a.	5	largest artery; conducts blood out of heart to rest of body
b.	4	returns deoxygenated blood to heart
c.	7	receives oxygenated blood from lungs
d.	8	pumps blood into body circulation
e.	6	takes blood to lungs
f.	9	carries blood to nephrons in kidney
g.	10	carries filtered blood back into circulation
h.	2	holding chamber for blood returned to heart
i.	3	pumps blood to lungs
j.	1	returns deoxygenated blood to heart
k.	11	carries urine to bladder

Matching II

Electrolytes	Abbreviation	Normal Serum Values
1. Bicarbonate	c	23–30
2. Calcium	a	8.6–10.3
3. Chloride	b	95–108
4. Magnesium	e	1.6–2.5
5. Phosphate	g	2.8–4.2
6. Potassium	d	3.5–5.2
7. Sodium	f	134–149

Matching III

Brand Names	Generic Names	Indica-tion	Type/Dosage Form
1.Aldactazide	j	D	diuretic combination
2. Aldactone	i	D	potassium-sparing diuretic
3. Demadex	k	D	loop diuretic
4. Diamox	a	D	carbonic anhy-drase inhibitor diuretic
5. Dyazide	l	D	diuretic combination
6. Kaon	h	P	oral liquid
7. K-dur	g	P	CR tablet
8. Klor-Con M	g	P	ER tablet
9. Klorvess	f	P	effervescent tablet
10. K-Tab	g	P	CR tablet
11. Lasix	d	D	loop diuretic
12. Maxzide	l	D	diuretic combination
13. Midamor	b	D	potassium-sparing diuretic
14. Moduretic	c	D	diuretic combination
15. Zaroxolyn	e	D	thiazide-like diuretic

True or False

1. **F**   The human heart has four chambers; two are ventricles and two are atria.

2. **T**

3. **T**

4. **F**   Veins have valves that prevent blood from flowing backward or pooling in the extremities.

5. **F**   The rate at which the water and solutes from the blood are filtered into the renal tubule is termed glomerular filtration rate (GFR).

6. **F**   Sodium is the most abundant cation in the body.

7. **F**   Anions carry a negative charge.

8. **T**

9. **T**

10. **F**   Hypertensive nephropathy refers to the kidney damage related to longstanding high blood pressure.

Short Answer

1. Coronary artery disease is characterized by the development of atherosclerotic plaques, accumulations of cholesterol, and cells that can block the flow of blood through the coronary arteries. If blood cannot reach the cardiac muscle cells, ischemia (deficiency of the blood supply) occurs resulting in a lack of oxygen and the death of a portion of the muscle, more commonly known as a heart attack.

2. Electrolyte homeostasis is the balance between and among electrolytes (such as K, Na, Ca, Cl, etc.) in the body— enough to perform body functions but not an excess, which could result in serious dysfunction. The kidneys maintain proper balance by holding on to the electrolytes the body needs while excreting those that are in excess.

3. Diuretics can deplete body potassium levels, leading to hypokalemia (which can cause life-threatening arrhythmias); potassium supplements are prescribed to prevent this.

4. pH is a measure of acidity, with a neutral pH being 7 (on a 0–14 scale), so the body's normal pH of about 7.4 is near neutral. Bicarbonate is important in maintaining the body's acid–base balance.

5. A kidney stone is a solid precipitate of substances the kidney should be reabsorbing or excreting, usually calcium oxalate. A kidney stone can cause pain as it travels through the urinary system, and, if it is too large to pass, it may cause an obstruction that blocks the flow of urine and possibly causing permanent kidney damage.

CHAPTER 14

Hypertension

Matching I

Brand Names	Generic Names	S, N, ISA, or M
1. Brevibloc	e	S
2. Bystolic	i	ISA
3. Coreg	d	M
4. Corgard	h	N
5. Inderal	j	N
6. InnoPran XL	j	N
7. Lopressor	g	S
8. Sectral	a	ISA
9. Tenormin	b	S
10. Toprol XL	g	S
11. Trandate	f	M
12. Zebeta	c	S

Matching II

Brand Names	Generic Names	Type (ACEI or ARB)
1. Accupril	j	ACEI
2. Aceon	i	ACEI
3. Altace	k	ACEI
4. Atacand	b	ARB
5. Avapro	d	ARB
6. Benicar	h	ARB
7. Cozaar	f	ARB
8. Diovan	n	ARB
9. Lotensin	a	ACEI
10. Mavik	m	ACEI
11. Micardis	l	ARB
12. Prinivil	e	ACEI
13. Univasc	g	ACEI
14. Vasotec	c	ACEI
15. Zestril	e	ACEI

Matching III

Brand Names	Generic Names	Class	Extended Release/ Injection
1. Adalat CC	h	CCB	ER
2. Calan SR	j	CCB	ER
3. Cardene	g	CCB	inj
4. Cardura XL	e	K	ER
5. Cartia XT	d	CCB	ER
6. Catapres	c	L	
7. Cleviprex	b	CCB	inj
8. Covera-HS	j	CCB	ER
9. Dilacor XR	d	CCB	ER
10. Nitropress	i	V	inj
11. Norvasc	a	CCB	
12. Procardia XL	h	CCB	ER
13. Tenex	f	L	
14. Tiazac	d	CCB	ER
15. Verelan PM	j	CCB	ER

Matching IV

Side Effects	Drug Class(es)
1. Angioedema	a
2. Asthma	d
3. Bradycardia	c, d, f
4. Congestive heart failure	c, d, f
5. Dizziness	a, b, c, d, e, f
6. Dry cough	a
7. Edema	e
8. Headache	e
9. Hyperglycemia	g
10. Hyperkalemia	a, b
11. Hyperuricemia	g
12. Impotence	c, d
13. Kidney failure	a, b
14. Orthostatic hypotension	a, b, e
15. Reflex tachycardia	e

True or False

1. **T**

2. **F** High blood pressure resulting from conditions such as kidney disease or hyperthyroidism is known as secondary hypertension.

3. **T**

4. **F** Medication treatment for hypertension is usually supplemented with lifestyle changes including diet, weight loss, and physical activity.

5. **F** Thiazide diuretics are usually considered first-line agents for treatment of hypertension.

6. **F** Cardioselective beta blockers have fewer side effects than nonselective blockers because they act on fewer body systems besides the cardiovascular system.

7. **T**

8. **T**

9. **F** Hypertrichosis, or excess hair growth, is a side effect of the antihypertensive minoxidil.

10. **F** When pregnant patients must be treated for hypertension, an alpha-2 agonist, methyldopa, is the drug of choice. ACEIs are contraindicated in pregnancy.

Short Answer

1. High blood pressure does not initially cause symptoms that are noticeable to patients, but over time, uncontrolled hypertension can result in damage to the kidneys, brain, heart, vasculature, and eyes, some of which can be life threatening.

2. Most hypertensive patients require multiple medications to control their disease; combinations can reduce the number of pills they take daily. The disadvantages are a reduction in flexibility for dose adjustments and frequently higher costs when generic combinations are not available.

3. The generic medications combined with hydrochlorothiazide (HCTZ) are Avalide and Hyzaar, which have the ARBs irbesartan and losartan; Prinzide and Zestoretic have the ACEI, lisinopril.

4. For patients without other issues, thiazides are chosen because they are inexpensive and have few side effects. When additional drugs are needed, they may be chosen based on the patients' other medical conditions. Those with CHF or a history of heart disease may get additional benefit from beta blockers or ACEIs. Patients with chest pain may have that reduced along with their blood pressure when they take CCBs. Patients with diabetes may have reduced risk of cardiovascular complications from their condition if they take ACEIs or ARBs.

5. Hypertensive crisis may be either urgency or emergency. Urgency is defined as blood pressure above 180/120 without signs of organ damage or failure and is treated with oral administration of captopril, labetalol, or clonidine. Hypertensive emergencies are situations where the blood pressure elevation is accompanied by signs of organ damage or failure and requires intravenous treatment with nitroprusside, clevidipine, and/or esmolol that are rapidly acting drugs, enabling a quick reduction of blood pressure, having a short duration of action, enabling fine-tuning of the dosage to control the patient's pressure, and reducing the incidence of side effects.

CHAPTER 15

Heart Disease

Matching I

Definitions	Terms	Abbrev.
1. Abnormal pattern of heart beats	b	
2. Blocked coronary arteries resulting in insufficient oxygen to heart	j	
3. Blocked coronary arteries resulting in myocardial cell death	k	MI
4. Bypass of blocked coronary arteries using blood vessels from patient's legs	f	CABG
5. Cardiac output insufficient for the body's needs	h	CHF
6. Graphic representation of heart's electrical activity	g	EKG
7. Insufficient blood flow resulting from damage to heart	e	
8. Life-threatening cardiovascular emergency	a	ACS
9. Placement of a stent to open blocked coronary arteries	l	PCI
10. Procedure to visualize and/or open blocked coronary arteries	d	
11. Relating to cardiac contractility	i	
12. Slower than normal heart rate	c	

Matching II

Brand Names	Generic Names	Class
1. Activase	b	CB
2. Aggrastat	j	GI
3. Ecotrin	c	AP
4. Fragmin	e	LMWH
5. Integrilin	g	GI
6. Lovenox	f	LMWH
7. Plavix	d	AP
8. ReoPro	a	GI
9. Retavase	h	CB
10. TNKase	i	CB

Matching III

Brand Names	Generic Names	Dosage	Long Acting
1. Dilatrate-SR	a	PC	LA
2. Imdur	b	PT	LA
3. Isordil	a	PT	
4. Minitran	c	TP	LA
5. Nitro-Bid	c	TO	
6. Nitro-Dur	c	TP	LA
7. Nitrolingual	c	TL	
8. Nitrostat	c	SL	
9. Nitro-Time	c	PC	LA

Matching IV

Brand Names	Generic Names	Route(s)	Type
1. Betapace	i	PO, IV	III
2. Calan	j	PO	IV
3. Cordarone	a	PO, IV	III
4. Corvert	f	IV	III
5. Multaq	d	PO	III
6. Norpace	b	PO	IA
7. Rythmol	h	PO	IC
8. Tambocor	e	PO	IC
9. Tikosyn	c	PO	III
10. Xylocaine	g	IV	IB

True or False

1. **F** Ischemic heart disease is often accompanied by chest pain symptoms (angina), but some patients, especially those with diabetes or certain nervous system disorders, may experience no symptoms whatsoever.

2. **T**

3. **T**

4. **F** The first goal that must be reached in patients suffering from an acute coronary syndrome is to return blood flow to the area of the heart being damaged by ischemia. If PCI or CABG are not available, patients may receive fibrinolytic therapy such as reteplase or alteplase to break down the blood clot to help restore blood supply to the heart.

5. **F** Quinidine is notorious for causing severe gastro-intestinal complaints including vomiting, diarrhea, and abdominal cramping. Procainamide has been implicated as a cause of systemic lupus erythematosus.

6. **F** Although lidocaine is effective in controlling ventricular arrhythmias, there is no product (oral OR injectable) available for outpatient use.

7. **T**

8. **T**

9. **F** Some fluids used in the treatment of shock, including albumin, hetastarch, and dextran, are sometimes known as colloids.

10. **T**

Short Answer

1. Sublingual nitroglycerin tablets must be dispensed only in their original, amber glass container. They should be protected from light and heat to retain their efficacy. Unused tablets should be discarded 6 months after the first time the bottle is opened; patient may need regular refill reminders, especially those with infrequent symptoms whose supply may go out of date before it is all used.

2. Because the effectiveness of fibrinolytics decreases with the time elapsed after the onset of the cardiovascular event, it is important that therapy be initiated as soon as possible. When used to treat stroke, the window is only 3 hours from the onset of symptoms.

3. Digoxin is thought to improve heart failure symptoms by blocking a number of the harmful proteins and hormones that cause ventricular remodeling. It is available generically, so is inexpensive; it is dosed only once daily and may reduce heart failure symptoms and the risk for hospitalization. It does not, however, improve survival and has serious side effects such as nausea, dizziness, bradycardia, or other arrhythmias.

4. A positive inotrope is a medication that increases heart contractility. Dobutamine is a beta-1 agonist and works by stimulating the beta receptors of the heart to increase contractility. Milrinone is a PDE3 inhibitor, which works by causing an increase in the concentration of calcium in the heart cells.

5. Medications most likely to be used in emergencies include vasopressors (drugs to increase blood pressure), including epinephrine and vasopressin, drugs to control heart rate (adenosine, atropine), and various antiarrhythmics (especially amiodarone, beta antagonists, diltiazem, and lidocaine). Additionally, most code kits or crash carts will include electrolytes such as calcium chloride and magnesium sulfate, along with concentrated (50%) dextrose injection.

CHAPTER 16

Hyperlipidemia

Matching I

Side/Adverse Effects	Class(es)
1. Bloating, belching	d
2. Blood glucose elevation	c
3. Constipation, flatulence	a
4. Fishy aftertaste	d
5. Flushing	c
6. Liver damage	b, c, e
7. Myalgia (muscle pain)	c
8. Nausea, vomiting, diarrhea, heartburn	e
9. Rhabdomyolysis	b, c, e
10. Upset stomach	b

Matching II

Brand Names	Generic Names	Class	Dosage Form(s)
1. Antara	f	fibrate	capsule
2. Colestid	d	bile acid sequestrant	powder, tablet
3. Crestor	m	statin	tablet
4. Lescol	h	statin	tablet
5. Lipitor	a	statin	tablet
6. Lipofen	f	fibrate	capsule
7. Livalo	k	statin	tablet
8. Lofibra	f	fibrate	tablet
9. Lopid	i	fibrate	tablet
10. Lovaza	g	omega 3	capsule
11. Mevacor	j	statin	tablet
12. Pravachol	l	statin	tablet
13. Prevalite	b	bile acid sequestrant	powder
14. Questran	b	bile acid sequestrant	powder
15. Tricor	f	fibrate	tablet

16. Triglide	**f**	fibrate	tablet
17. Trilipix	**f**	fibrate	capsule
18. Welchol	**c**	bile acid sequestrant	tablet
19. Zetia	**e**	cholesterol absorption inhibitor	tablet
20. Zocor	**n**	statin	tablet

True or False

1. **F** One of the many types of lipids in the human body can be classified as cholesterol. Others include phospholipids and the fat-soluble vitamins A, D, E, and K.

2. **T**

3. **F** HDL (high density lipoprotein) is known as good cholesterol because elevated levels are associated with a lower risk of developing heart disease. OR LDL (low density lipoprotein) is known as bad cholesterol because elevated levels are associated with a higher risk of developing heart disease.

4. **F** Cholesterol and triglyceride concentrations in the blood reflect those that are consumed in the diet and also those that are produced by the body.

5. **T**

6. **T**

7. **T**

8. **F** The many different formulations of fenofibrate have slightly different doses and release mechanisms so they are not interchangeable.

9. **F** Ezetimibe is classified as a cholesterol absorption inhibitor.

10. **F** Omega 3 fatty acids may lower triglyceride levels by as much as 50%.

Short Answer

1. The TLC Diet recommends that less than 7% of calories come from saturated fat and substitutes lean meats and skim milk for beef and whole milk, restricts cholesterol intake, and increases mono- and poly-unsaturated fats. Other recommendations include increasing soluble fiber and plant sterols and stanols such as those in soybeans.

2. The pleiotropic effects of statins include reduction of inflammation and stabilization of atherosclerotic plaques, making them more organized and less likely to rupture.

3. Sustained-release niacin allows patients to take their doses twice daily instead of the TID (three times daily) regimen required with the immediate-release product. Although the sustained-release formulations reduce the flushing side effect of the immediate-release dosage forms, they are accompanied by a significant increase in the risk of liver damage.

4. For most patients, therapy with ezetimibe yields a modest 18% reduction in circulating LDL particles. Because of this relatively small decrease in LDL, a lack of studies showing an improvement in cardiovascular risk, and no significant effect on other parts of the lipid profile, ezetimibe is usually used as an adjunctive treatment for patients unable to meet their cholesterol goals on other hyperlipidemia treatments for patients who cannot tolerate statins due to adverse events.

5. It is generally recommended that patients take other medications at least 1 hour before or 4–6 hours after the bile acid sequestrant doses because bile acid sequestrants may bind other drugs in the gastrointestinal tract, interfering with their absorption.

CHAPTER 17

Overview of the Respiratory System

Matching I

Part	Letter	Function
1. Alveoli	i	gas exchange
2. Bronchiole	e	branch of the bronchus, carrying air to alveoli
3. Bronchus	d	branch of the trachea, carrying air deeper into the lung
4. Diaphragm	f	primary muscle of respiration
5. Lung	c	primary respiratory organ
6. Pharynx	f	connects nose and mouth
7. Pulmonary artery	g	delivers blood to the lung
8. Pulmonary vein	h	carries oxygenated blood away from the lung
9. Trachea	b	passageway for air into the lung

Matching II

Definitions	Terms	Abbreviation
1. Amount of air exhaled with force after maximum inhalation	c	FVC
2. Device that delivers aerosolized medication to the lungs	d	MDI
3. Device to deliver medications to the lungs as a fine mist using a compressor	e	
4. Device used to deliver medication to the lungs without an aerosol propellant	b	DPI
5. Measure of oxygen and carbon dioxide in the blood	a	ABG
6. Tests of lung function	f	PFTs
7. Tube which connects to the mouthpiece of an inhaler to increase the amount of medication reaching the lungs	g	

True or False

1. **T**

2. **F** Carbon dioxide is a waste product of cellular metabolism.

3. **T**

4. **F** Nebulizers are often used by pediatric and elderly populations as they do not require good coordination for proper medication administration the way MDIs and DPIs do.

5. **F** DPIs should be discarded 30 days after the sealed pouch in which they are dispensed is opened.

6. **T**

7. **F** Spacers are often recommended to increase the amount of drug the patient will take into the lungs.

8. **F** Metered dose inhalers should be primed before the first use by expelling one dose.

9. **T**

10. **F** Nebulizers usually require electricity from an outlet or battery to deliver medication.

Short Answer

1. Inhalation is the preferred method of medication administration for the treatment of most pulmonary conditions because the medication is rapidly deposited and absorbed for action directly where it is needed, providing faster symptom relief. Additionally, the specificity of inhaled medication for the lungs also decreases the likelihood of systemic (body-wide) adverse effects.

2. Patients using an inhaled corticosteroid should rinse their mouths after each use to prevent irritation or possible infection.

3. MDIs should be cleaned at least once a week by removing the canister and rinsing the mouthpiece with warm water. Spacers should also be cleaned weekly in warm water with a drop of liquid dish soap.

CHAPTER 18

Disorders of the Respiratory System

Matching I

Brand Names	Generic Names	Route	Indication(s)	Dosage Form
1. Accolate	m	O	A	oral
2. Aerobid	d	P	A	inhaled (MDI)
3. Asmanex	h	P	A	inhaled (DPI)
4. Atrovent	f	P	COPD	inhaled (MDI)
5. Flovent	e	P	A	inhaled (MDI)
6. ProAir HFA	a	P	A, COPD	inhaled (MDI)
7. Pulmicort	c	P	A	inhaled (DPI)
8. QVAR	b	P	A	inhaled (MDI)
9. Serevent	k	P	A, COPD	inhaled (DPI)
10. Singulair	i	O	A	oral
11. Spiriva	l	P	COPD	inhaled (DPI)
12. Ventolin HFA	a	P	A, COPD	inhaled (MDI)
13. Xolair	j	Q	A	subcutaneous
14. Xopenex	g	P	A	inhaled (Neb)
15. Zyflo	n	O	A	oral

Fill-In

Brand Names	Beta Agonist	Other Ingredient	Category
1. Advair	salmeterol	fluticasone	ICS
2. Combivent	albuterol	ipratropium	anticholinergic
3. Dulera	formoterol	mometasone	ICS
4. Symbicort	formoterol	budesonide	ICS

True or False

1. **F** Patients with asthma and COPD should receive yearly immunizations against influenza and be sure they are up to date on their other immunizations. (Pneumonia vaccine is longlasting and is seldom given more than once.)
2. **T**
3. **F** Acute asthma is the term used for severe asthma symptoms that can progress quickly to an emergent, potentially fatal situation.
4. **T**
5. **F** Inhaled corticosteroids may be used alone or as part of combination therapy for the treatment of asthma and are never considered for use as rescue medications.
6. **T**
7. **T**
8. **F** Inhaled corticosteroids should not be used as therapy for the treatment of COPD.
9. **T**
10. **F** Cystic fibrosis patients often require higher doses of antibiotics because they typically have a faster clearance rate than patients without CF.

Short Answer

1. The typical course for asthma is an intense period of exacerbation in which symptoms are increased followed by periods of remission, when symptoms are minimal or nonexistent.

2. The time between exacerbation and remission is variable and generally depends on asthma control. An exacerbation may be brought on by an environmental trigger such as an allergen, virus, pollution, or tobacco smoke.

3. Quick-relief medications, also known as rescue medications, are fast-acting agents taken on an as-needed basis and only for immediate relief of an asthma exacerbation.

4. The main action of beta 2-agonists is relaxation of the smooth muscles of the lung airways, resulting in dilation of the airways and relief of bronchoconstriction. SABAs are appropriate treatment for as needed relief of acute exacerbations for all stages of COPD, but frequent dosing inhibits their usefulness as a daily therapy. The inhalation preparation of SABA is preferred over oral and parenteral forms as all preparations have equivalent efficacy, but the specificity of inhalation preparation to the lungs results in decreased side effects. LABA are appropriate for COPD symptom reduction in a convenient, twice daily dosing schedule.

5. Pancreatic enzyme deficiency is a common difficulty in patients with cystic fibrosis because thick mucus plugs the pancreatic ducts and blocks the release of pancreatic enzymes needed for the digestion of fat and protein and the absorption of vitamins A, D, E, and K (fat soluble vitamins). Without these pancreatic enzymes, malnutrition will occur. The signs and symptoms of decreased pancreatic enzymes are abdominal distension, foul-smelling loose bowel movement, flatulence, and malnourishment. Cystic fibrosis patients must replace the pancreatic enzymes to ensure proper nutrition and normal growth.

CHAPTER 19

Acid-Related Diseases of the Upper Gastrointestinal Tract

Matching I

Brand Names	Generic Names	Class	OTC?
1. Aciphex	i	PPI	N
2. Axid AR	f	H2RA	Y
3. Dexilant	b	PPI	N
4. Nexium	c	PPI	N
5. Pepcid AC	d	H2RA	Y
6. Prevacid 24HR	e	PPI	Y
7. Prilosec	g	PPI	Y
8. Protonix	h	PPI	N
9. Tagamet HB	a	H2RA	Y
10. Zantac-150	j	H2RA	Y

Matching II

Conditions	Definition	OTC or Referral
1. Dyspepsia	d	OTC
2. Gastroesophageal reflux disease	c	OTC
3. Peptic ulcer disease	b	referral
4. Stress-related mucosal damage	a	referral

True or False

1. **F**   Antacids work by reacting with stomach acid to neutralize it.

2. **T**

3. **T**

4. **F**   Proton pump inhibitors work by inhibiting gastric acid secretion.

5. **T**

6. **F**   Liquid bismuth preparations can cause blackening of the tongue and stools.

7. **F**   Eradication of *H. pylori* and ulcer-healing requires treatment with at least three different drugs, including one to inhibit acid secretion and two antibiotics.

8. **T**

9. **T**

10. **F**   Patients with one of the three primary risk factors for SRMB (intubation, blood clotting disruption, or sepsis) should have SRMB prophylaxis started immediately.

Short Answer

1. The upper gastrointestinal (UGI) tract begins with the mouth and ends in the small intestine at the junction of the duodenum and jejunum. The esophagus is a muscular tube, which lies behind the heart and connects the oropharynx to the stomach. The lower esophageal sphincter (LES) is a valve that guards against stomach contents from refluxing back into the esophagus. When the sphincter relaxes, it permits food to empty into the stomach. The stomach receives food, beverages, and medications from the esophagus, aids in digestion, and delivers these substances to the small intestine. The duodenum extends from the pylorus to the jejunum where the UGI tract ends and the lower GI tract begins. The pylorus regulates the passage of partially digested foods and other substances into the duodenum and acts like a sphincter, which guards the opening between the stomach antrum and the duodenum.

2. Medications used to treat acid-related UGI diseases are divided into two groups: drugs that decrease stomach acidity and drugs that work by mechanisms that do not alter stomach acid. Antacids, the histamine 2-receptor antagonists, and the proton pump inhibitors all decrease stomach acidity and, thus, increase stomach pH. Sucralfate, bismuth salts, misoprostol, and alginic acid all provide benefits without altering stomach acid.

3. For the best effect, it is recommended that patients take a PPI 30–60 minutes prior to eating. The PPIs work best when taken before a meal so that the proton pumps are actively secreting acid.

4. Nonsteroidal anti-inflammatory drugs (NSAIDs) can cause peptic ulcers. These drugs act directly on the stomach lining to cause erosions, but ulcers (which are deeper than erosions) are related to the ability of the NSAID to systemically inhibit naturally occurring protective prostaglandins in the stomach lining.

5. Patients with bleeding peptic ulcers usually present with vomiting of blood; bloody or dark, tarry stools (melena); or both. Patients with SRMB may present with small amounts of blood in the stomach contents when a nasogastric tube is being used for feedings or medication administration, or small amounts of blood may be identified in stool samples that are tested for its presence. Others may present with large amounts

of blood or coffee ground-like material in the patient's vomit, in nasogastric aspirates, or with bloody diarrhea. Patients with these signs or symptoms represent a medical emergency that must be dealt with immediately as these patients can quickly go into hypovolemic shock (cardiovascular instability caused by a substantial loss in blood volume).

CHAPTER 20

Nausea, Vomiting, and Upper GI Tract Motility Disorders

Matching

Brand Names	Generic Names	Status	Route(s)
1. Aloxi	i	RX	IV
2. Antivert	e	OTC	PO
3. Anzemet	c	RX	IV
4. Cesamet	g	RX	PO
5. Compazine	k	RX	PO, PR, IV, IM
6. Dramamine	b	OTC	PO
7. Emend	a	RX	PO
8. Emetrol	j	OTC	PO
9. Marinol	d	RX	PO
10. Phenergan	l	RX	PO, PR, IV, IM, TD
11. Reglan	f	RX	PO, IV
12. Tigan	n	RX	PO, IM
13. Transderm Scōp	m	RX	TD
14. Zofran	h	RX	PO, IV

True or False

1. **F** Patients whose vomiting is caused by more difficult to manage issues such as chemotherapy or diabetic gastroparesis may become dehydrated and develop electrolyte imbalances and weight loss.

2. **T**

3. **T**

4. **F** Cannabinoid antiemetics are controlled substances because they are chemically related to the principle active ingredient of marijuana.

5. **F** Patients whose nausea and vomiting are accompanied by fever and diarrhea should be referred to their primary care providers or an emergency department for further evaluation.

6. **F** Chamomile (Matricaria recutita) and peppermint oil (Mentha piperita) are both thought to have antispasmodic properties that may reduce nausea, and both are labeled GRAS (generally recognized as safe by FDA) status in the United States.

7. **T**

8. **T**

9. **F** People who are vomiting because of motion sickness may not be able to keep down an oral product and absorb medication from it; a transdermal patch may be a better remedy.

10. **T**

Short Answer

1. GI diseases can cause nausea and vomiting as well as other types of disorders (including cardiovascular, infectious, neurologic, or metabolic disease). Certain medications (particularly medications associated with the treatment of cancer), as well as conditions such as pregnancy, postoperative states, motion sickness, and motility disorders can also cause nausea and vomiting.

2. Chemotherapy-induced nausea and vomiting (CINV) can be divided into three categories: acute, delayed, and anticipatory. Acute CINV occurs within 24 hours after receiving chemotherapy, while delayed occurs more than 24 hours after the therapy. Anticipatory nausea and vomiting happens before the chemotherapy dose in some patients who have experienced acute or delayed nausea and vomiting previously.

3. When choosing a treatment for a pregnant patient suffering from nausea and vomiting, teratogenic potential should be of primary concern. Nonpharmacologic alternatives, such as behavioral, dietary, and physical modifications, should be considered first. Drugs that have been used and are considered to be safe during pregnancy include pyridoxine, doxylamine, promethazine, metoclopramide, and trimethobenzamide. Methylprednisolone is a corticosteroid that may be considered for nausea and vomiting of pregnancy, but it has been associated with birth defects if used during the first trimester. Risks versus benefits must be weighed in all situations.

4. Gastroparesis can present in some patients as nausea, vomiting, bloating, constipation, or diarrhea. It is commonly seen in poorly controlled diabetic patients who have autonomic neuropathy.

5. Patients who are experiencing simple nausea/vomiting from gastritis or another self-limiting illness will probably benefit from nonpharmacological or OTC products initially. Patients who are traveling and have problems with motion sickness may also receive effective treatment with OTC products like diphenhydramine and meclizine.

CHAPTER 21

Lower Gastrointestinal Tract

Matching I

Brand Names	Generic Names	Indication	Status
1. Benefiber	g	C	OTC
2. Colace	d	C	OTC
3. Dulcolax	a	C	OTC
4. Enulose	e	C	RX
5. Ex-Lax	j	C	OTC
6. Haley's M-O	k	C	OTC
7. Imodium	f	D	OTC
8. Konsyl	i	C	OTC
9. Kristalose	e	C	RX
10. Lomotil	c	D	RX
11. Maltsupex	g	C	OTC
12. Metamucil	i	C	OTC
13. MiraLAX	h	C	OTC
14. Pepto Bismol	b	D	OTC
15. Senokot	j	C	OTC

Matching II

Brand Names	Generic Names	Indication
1. Asacol	f	L
2. Azulfidine	j	L
3. Cimzia	d	L
4. Colazal	c	L
5. Dipentum	h	L
6. Humira	a	L
7. Lotronex	b	M
8. Mylicon	i	K
9. Pentasa	f	L
10. Remicade	e	L
11. Rowasa	f	L
12. Tysabri	g	L

True or False

1. **F** The most important treatment for acute diarrhea is preventing dehydration. (Most cases of acute diarrhea are self-limiting and may not require ANY medication.)

2. **F** Loperamide in any dosage form should not be given to children under 2 years of age.

3. **T**

4. **T**

5. **T**

6. **F** Patients taking opioid medication for cancer pain often require laxatives to maintain regular bowel function.

7. **F** Non-saline hyperosmotic laxatives stimulate defecation by drawing water into the bowel and promote local irritation, stimulating evacuation. Stool softeners may be taken for constipation and draw water into the bowel but are not considered laxatives.

8. **T**

9. **F** Irritable bowel syndrome and inflammatory bowel disease are different conditions, with different causes and treatments.

10. **F** Patients who are allergic to sulfonamides (sulfa) are likely to also be allergic to sulfasalazine; mesalamine does not have the sulfonamide molecule as part of the drug.

Short Answer

1. Probiotics are dietary supplements of live microorganisms which, when administered in adequate amounts, confer a health benefit. The most common species useful in the treatment or prevention of acute, uncomplicated diarrhea is *Lactobacillus acidophilus*, a type of bacteria that normally live in the human small intestine and vagina. Because *Lactobacillus* is naturally occurring bacteria in the lower gastrointestinal tract, it is useful in the restoration and stabilization of the normal intestinal flora (harmless microorganisms that inhabit the intestinal tract and are essential for its normal functioning). *Lactobacillus* also interferes with the ability of pathogenic bacteria to adhere (attach) to intestinal mucosal cells and establish an infection.

2. Psyllium and other bulk-forming laxatives must be taken with at least a full glass of water or other liquid either before or after meals. Without adequate fluid, the product can swell and block the throat or esophagus, which could lead to choking. Patients who have difficulty swallowing should not take these products.

3. Because inflammatory bowel disease and rheumatoid arthritis are both autoimmune disorders, the monoclonal antibodies that are therapies for joint disease because they target receptors in the immune system may also be effective for Crohn's disease and ulcerative colitis.

4. Alosetron is indicated only for irritable bowel syndrome (IBS) with diarrhea, but, in the past, was sometimes prescribed for diarrhea caused by other conditions, resulting in serious and fatal side effects. The Prescribing Program for Lotronex (PPL) requires a physician to undergo training to monitor the medication and its effects. Pharmacy technicians should remember that every prescription written for Lotronex must have a safety sticker affixed to the paper prescription and that prescriptions for alosetron may not be transmitted verbally, by phone, or electronically (via fax or computer). FDA requires a medication guide each time the drug is dispensed.

5. Treatments that help eliminate worms from the body usually work in one of two ways. They either attack the adult worm, or they inhibit the ability of the eggs to form and grow, terminating the life cycle. These mechanisms support the pulse therapy (short bursts of medications) that is common with antiparasite treatment.

CHAPTER 22

Hepatic and Pancreatic Disorders

Matching I

Definitions	Terms
1. Abdominal organ responsible for synthesizing proteins, cholesterol, and bile	g
2. Abnormal accumulation of fluid in the abdominal cavity	a
3. Brain/nervous system dysfunction caused by ammonia and waste products in the blood	d
4. Enlarged veins in the upper GI tract, which may burst and bleed easily	l
5. Increased pressure in the main vein of the liver	j
6. Infection of ascitic fluid in the peritoneal cavity	k
7. Inflammation of the liver	e
8. Inflammation of the pancreas	i
9. Liver disease in which scar tissue replaces normal tissue	c
10. Organ that secretes insulin, glucagon, somatostatin, and some digestive enzymes	h
11. Substance that helps remove fat-soluble substances from the body and aids in intestinal fat absorption	b
12. Yellow discoloration of skin and eyes caused by bilirubin accumulation	f

Matching II

Brand Names	Generic Names	Disease Type	Condition
1. Aldactone	i	L	ascites
2. Creon	f	P	malabsorption
3. Enulose	b	L	hepatic encephalopathy
4. Inderal LA	g	L	variceal bleeding
5. Lasix	a	L	ascites
6. Neo-Fradin	c	L	hepatic encephalopathy
7. Noroxin	d	L	SBP
8. Sandostatin	e	L	variceal bleeding
9. Xifaxan	h	L	hepatic encephalopathy
10. Zenpep	f	P	malabsorption

True or False

1. **T**

2. **F** Variceal bleeding is the term used to refer to bleeding from surface vessels in the upper GI tract that have become enlarged due to the increased pressure in the portal vein that results from cirrhosis.

3. **F** The most common diuretic regimen for treating ascites is a combination of furosemide with a potassium-sparing diuretic, usually spironolactone.

4. **T**

5. **T**

6. **F** Rifaximin is as effective as lactulose, neomycin, and metronidazole for the treatment of SBP but is much more expensive.

7. **T**

8. **F** Albumin infusions can help maintain blood volume and prevent kidney disorders in patients with liver disease.

9. **F** Pancreatic enzymes are administered orally.

10. **T**

Short Answer

1. The major complications of cirrhosis include ascites, hepatic encephalopathy, spontaneous bacterial peritonitis, and variceal bleeding.

2. For hospitalized patients who cannot swallow, 300 mL of lactulose may be mixed with 700 mL of water and administered as a retention enema (retained in the colon for least 1 hour).

3. Patients who develop an acute episode of SBP are typically hospitalized and require systemic IV antibiotic treatment as initial therapy for a total of 5 days. This is most often a third generation cephalosporin, such as ceftriaxone or cefotaxime as initial therapy. Alternatives include fluoroquinolones, such as ciprofloxacin or levofloxacin, or extended spectrum penicillins, such as ampicillin/sulbactam, which are also effective.

4. The major obstacle to use of albumin is that it is very costly. A treatment course used for SBP or for paracentesis may cost several hundred dollars.

5. Pancreatic enzyme doses above the recommended maximum daily dose of 10,000 units/kg/day have been associated with inflammation and scarring of the inside of the intestinal tract, a condition known as fibrosing colonopathy.

CHAPTER 23

Nutritional Pharmacology

Matching

Terms	Definitions
1. Building blocks of body tissues, composed of amino acid combinations	e
2. Class of nutrients that includes sugar, starch, and fiber	a
3. Class of substances that includes fats, phospholipids, and cholesterol	c
4. Essential nutrients needed in small amounts for body functions	h
5. Fats that are solid at room temperature	f
6. Form of fat with a glycerol base on which three fatty acids are attached	g
7. Inorganic elements used for body processes	d
8. Non-nutrient lipid made by (and present in) humans and animals, but not plants	b

Fill-In

Vitamins	Letter/Number	Type
Biotin	B7	W
Alpha tocopherol	E	F
Ascorbic acid	C	W
Beta carotene	A	F
Calcitriol	D	F
Cholecalciferol	D	F
Cyanocobalamin	B12	W
Ergocalciferol	D	F
Hydroxocobalamin	B12	W
Niacin	B3	W
Pantothenic acid	B5	W
Phytonadione	K	F
Pyridoxine	B6	W
Retinol	A	F
Riboflavin	B2	W
Thiamine	B1	W

True or False

1. **T**

2. **F** Patients should be advised to choose the vitamin supplement that best matches their specific nutrient needs.

3. **T**

4. **F** Although vitamin supplements are natural dietary products, they should be included on a patient's medication profile so that they can be screened for interactions.

5. **T**

6. **F** Parenteral nutrition is a nutrient preparation administered intravenously; enteral nutrition is administered via the gastrointestinal tract.

7. **T**

8. **F** The protein source for most parenteral nutrition is amino acid solution.

9. **F** Natural weight loss products, such as guarana extract and chromium picolinate, have not been studied extensively enough to have a documented recommended dosage and are not endorsed or regulated by the FDA.

10. **T**

Short Answer

1. The National Institutes of Health suggest that people who might benefit from multiple vitamin and mineral supplementation include postmenopausal women (calcium with vitamin D), women of childbearing age (folic acid), people over the age of 50 (vitamin B12), pregnant women (iron), and breastfed infants (vitamin D), as well as those with poor dietary nutrient intake, patients on restricted (e.g., vegan) or low-calorie diets, and those with medical conditions that interfere with absorption or use of nutrients.

2. Because many multiple vitamin supplements contain the full recommended dietary allowance of several ingredients, it is possible that people who take them regularly could exceed the recommended maximum levels for those nutrients. Additionally, some vitamin supplements can interfere with medication therapy.

3. Some patients for whom nutrition support may be necessary include those who are unable to fulfill their nutritional needs by consuming food because of illness, decreased appetite, difficulty swallowing, or surgery that interferes with eating.

4. Cycling is the infusion of a full day's worth of TPN over a shorter time period than 24 hours. Advantages of this include giving the patient time to be free of tubing and pumps for increased movement, especially if going to school or work, and a recovery period for the liver to prevent long-term damage.

5. The FDA has approved a lipase inhibitor, orlistat, to decrease caloric intake by preventing absorption of dietary fat. It has also approved some appetite suppressants (anorexiants), including benzphetamine, diethylpropion, phendimetrazine, and phentermine.

CHAPTER 24

Overview of the Hematologic System

Matching I

Terms	Definitions
1. Blood cell protein that carries oxygen	g
2. Blood cell responsible for forming clots	l
3. Decreased number of white blood cells	i
4. Growth factor controlling production of red blood cells	e
5. Liquid component of blood	k
6. Mature red blood cell	d
7. Most common protein in plasma	a
8. Process of forming a blood clot	c
9. Storage form of iron in the blood	f
10. Substance that provokes the immune system	b
11. Type of white blood cell that responds to infectious agents	j
12. White blood cell	h

True or False

1. **F** A lymphocyte is a white blood cell.

2. **T**

3. **T**

4. **F** The recommended daily allowance (RDA) of iron varies by age, sex, and pregnancy status.

5. **T**

6. **F** Hemoglobin levels show the existence of anemia but not its cause.

7. **F** White blood cells usually increase in number when a patient has a bacterial infection.

8. **T**

9. **F** Smokers tend to have higher levels of hemoglobin than nonsmokers.

10. **T**

Short Answer

1. Blood consists of fluid (plasma) and formed elements (cell fragments and cells). The cells are suspended within the plasma. The cells include red blood cells (RBCs) or erythrocytes, white blood cells (WBCs) or leukocytes, and platelets (thrombocytes).

2. The body depends on the hemoglobin in the blood to deliver oxygen, and the hemoglobin molecule has four iron ions, so iron is an essential part of it. If iron supplies cannot meet the demand of RBC production, small, pale RBCs will be formed that will not carry oxygen efficiently and may cause symptoms of an iron deficiency anemia.

3. Hemostasis is made up of three important steps: a narrowing of the damaged blood vessel known as vasoconstriction, the formation of a platelet plug, and the formation of a blood clot through the clotting cascade.

4. Vitamin K is essential to the production of clotting factors II, VII, IX, and X. If the body's stores are low, the production of these factors will decrease and clot formation will be more difficult to achieve, increasing the risk of bleeding. Warfarin interferes with vitamin K, preventing unwanted/unneeded coagulation.

5. The WBCs are responsible for defending the body from infection. When a pathogen enters the body, neutrophils are the first cells to respond. They attack the invader and try to engulf it while sending out signals to attract other WBCs. Monocytes and their counterparts in the tissues, the macrophages, arrive next and also swallow pathogens. Lymphocytes are broken down into two groups. The T lymphocyte helps the body fight viral infections and kills off tumor cells. B lymphocytes, once activated, produce antibodies against antigens.

CHAPTER 25

Disorders of the Hematologic System

Matching I

Brand Names	Generic Names	I or ESA
1. Aranesp	a	ESA
2. DexFerrum	d	I
3. Epogen	b	ESA
4. Feraheme	c	I
5. Ferrlecit	f	I
6. InFeD	d	I
7. Procrit	b	ESA
8. Venofer	e	I

Matching II

Brand Names	Generic Names	Class	Route
1. Angiomax	a	T	IV
2. Arixtra	e	X	SQ
3. Coumadin	g	K	PO
4. Fragmin	c	L	SQ
5. Lovenox	d	L	SQ
6. Pradaxa	b	T	PO
7. Xarelto	f	X	PO

True or False

1. **F** Macrocytic anemia must be treated with both folic acid and vitamin B12 to address all the effects of the disease.

2. **T**

3. **F** Patients who have been affected by heparin-induced thrombocytopenia (HIT) should not receive future heparin therapy but can be treated with thrombin inhibitors or Factor Xa inhibitors if they require anticoagulants.

4. **F** Low molecular weight heparins (LMWHs) have a longer duration of action than unfractionated heparin and must be administered less frequently.

5. **T**

6. **F** Dabigatran therapy requires fewer laboratory tests and dosage adjustments than warfarin therapy.

7. **T**

8. **F** Vitamin K can be administered orally to reverse the anticoagulant actions of warfarin but not dabigatran.

9. **T**

10. **T**

Short Answer

1. Iron deficiency is a result of an underlying cause that must be corrected to treat the anemia properly. If the iron deficiency is a result of insufficient iron in the diet, iron supplementation alone may solve the problem; however, if the iron deficiency resulted from gastrointestinal bleeding or other type of hemorrhage, the cause of the bleeding must be treated as well.

2. Ferrous fumarate is 33% elemental iron, meaning that 100 mg of ferrous fumarate yields 33 mg of elemental iron. 200 mg/33 = approximately 6; 6 x 100 mg = 600 mg of ferrous fumarate would give a dose of 200 mg elemental iron.

3. Many types of drugs including antithyroid preparations, anti-inflammatories, psychotropics, anti-infectives, anticonvulsants, and diuretics may cause neutropenia. Cancer chemotherapy drugs are especially dangerous in this regard. Patients at risk of drug-induced neutropenia may be treated with the granulocyte colony stimulating factors (G-CSFs) filgrastim and pegfilgrastim to help prevent this adverse effect.

4. Heparin is indicated for prevention and treatment of deep vein thrombosis (DVT), pulmonary embolism (PE), heart attack, and stroke. It is also used to prevent clot formation during surgery, dialysis, and blood transfusions. It may be administered intravenously by continuous infusion or intermittent injection, as well as subcutaneously, depending on the reason for its use.

5. Because warfarin doses must be fine-tuned for each individual patient, issues like drug interactions and patient compliance become extremely important. Warfarin has many drug interactions, so the pharmacist must review the patient profile frequently to screen for any potential problems. Warfarin's action is dependent on antagonizing vitamin K, so patients must receive information about keeping their intake of this vitamin (from dietary sources like green leafy vegetables and any multiple vitamin products they take) consistent so that their anticoagulation stays within therapeutic limits.

CHAPTER 26

Bacterial Infections

Matching I

Brand Names	Generic Names	Routes	Class
1. Augmentin	b	X	aminopenicillin
2. Azactam	d	Z	monobactam
3. Bactocill	t	Z	antistaphylococcal
4. Bicillin LA	u	Z	natural
5. Cedax	k	X	3rd gen cephalosporin
6. Ceftin	m	X	2nd gen cephalosporin
7. Claforan	g	Z	3rd gen cephalosporin
8. Doribax	o	Z	carbapenem
9. Fortaz	j	Z	3rd gen cephalosporin
10. Invanz	p	Z	carbapenem
11. Keflex	n	X	1st gen cephalosporin
12. Mefoxin	h	Z	cephamycin
13. Merrem	r	Z	carbapenem
14. Moxatag	a	X	aminopenicillin
15. Nallpen	s	Z	antistaphylococcal
16. Primaxin	q	Z	carbapenem
17. Rocephin	l	Z	3rd gen cephalosporin
18. Spectracef	e	X	3rd gen cephalosporin
19. Suprax	f	X	3rd gen cephalosporin
20. Tazicef	j	Z	3rd gen cephalosporin
21. Teflaro	i	Z	5th gen cephalosporin
22. Timentin	w	Z	extended-spectrum penicillin
23. Unasyn	c	Z	aminopenicillin

24. Zinacef	m	Z	2nd gen cephalosporin
25. Zosyn	v	Z	extended-spectrum penicillin

Matching II

Brand Names	Generic Names	Class	Route of Administration
1. Akne-Mycin	d	M	Topical
2. Avelox	h	Q	IV, PO
3. Biaxin	c	M	PO
4. Cetraxal	b	Q	Otic
5. Ciloxan	b	Q	Ophthalmic
6. Cipro	b	Q	IV, PO
7. Dificid	e	M	PO
8. E.E.S.	d	M	PO
9. Erythrocin lactobionate	d	M	IV
10. Factive	f	Q	PO
11. Ilotycin	d	M	Ophthalmic
12. Iquix	g	Q	Ophthalmic
13. Levaquin	g	Q	IV, PO
14. Noroxin	i	Q	PO
15. Ocuflox	j	Q	Ophthalmic
16. PCE	d	M	PO
17. ProQuin XR	b	Q	PO
18. Quixin	g	Q	Ophthalmic
19. Zithromax	a	M	IV, PO
20. Zmax	a	M	PO

Matching III

Brand Names	Generic Names	Route(s)	Class
1. Bactrim	c	X	sulfonamide
2. Bleph-10	o	Y	sulfonamide
3. Cleocin	a	XZ	lincosamide
4. Coly-Mycin M	b	Z	cationic detergent

5. Cubicin	e	Z	lipopeptide
6. Doryx	f	X	tetracycline
7. Flagyl	i	XZ	bacteriostatic
8. Furadantin	k	X	miscellaneous
9. Macrobid	k	X	bactericidal
10. Minocin	j	XZ	tetracycline
11. Myambutol	g	X	antituberculosis
12. Rifadin	m	XZ	antituberculosis
13. Septra	c	X	sulfonamide
14. Seromycin	d	X	antituberculosis
15. Solodyn	j	X	tetracycline
16. Synercid	l	Z	streptogramin
17. Tygacil	p	Z	tetracycline
18. Vibramycin	f	X	tetracycline
19. Xifaxan	n	X	miscellaneous
20. Zyvox	h	XZ	oxazolidinone

True or False

1. **F** Some bacteria in the human body, called normal flora, do not cause harm or infection and protect the body against disease-causing organisms.

2. **F** Nosocomial is a term that refers to hospital-acquired or other healthcare-associated infections.

3. **T**

4. **F** Reserving broad-spectrum antibiotics for use only when other treatments will not cover the infection reduces the chance of development of antibiotic-resistant bacteria.

5. **T**

6. **F** Cephalosporins are not a good type of antibiotic to use for patients who have had a serious or life-threatening allergic reaction to a penicillin because they may have a similar reaction, but they may be administered to patients who have had a less severe allergic reaction.

7. **T**

8. **T**

9. **F** Linezolid is a drug that is effective against many resistant gram positive organisms and may be given intravenously or orally, but it is relatively expensive.

10. **T**

Short Answer

1. Samples of body materials such as blood, tissue, sputum, or urine are collected from patients suspected of having infections. Microscopic inspection can identify the shape of any bacteria they contain, and gram staining can categorize the organisms as gram positive or gram negative. Allowing the samples to grow in culture media and exposing them to specific antibiotics can enable the best choice of antibiotic for an infection.

2. Susceptibility refers to the sensitivity of a microorganism to a particular antibiotic and indicates the likelihood that an infection will respond to particular antibiotic therapy.

3. Aminoglycoside antibiotics are considered to have a narrow therapeutic window because, while patients must be given a high enough dose to achieve effective concentrations to treat their infections, too high a concentration can cause serious adverse effects. Because of the narrow therapeutic window, aminoglycoside serum levels are often ordered to indicate the maximum and minimum concentrations achieved.

4. All classes of penicillins have the same adverse effects and reactions, which include anaphylaxis, drug-fever, serum sickness, rash, nephritis, hemolytic anemia, and leucopenia. Side effects patients may experience when taking these medications include diarrhea, colitis, nausea, and vomiting. Hypersensitivity reactions are the most common adverse effect of cephalosporins (urticaria and anaphylaxis are rare). Many patients complain of pain with IM injections. Thrombophlebitis (inflammation of the vein) after IV use is possible. All cephalosporins can produce leukopenia and thrombocytopenia, and prolonged use can contribute to the development of *Clostridium difficile* (pseudomembranous) colitis. Fluoroquinolones can cause nausea, vomiting, and diarrhea as well as altered mental status and confusion when not properly adjusted for renal function. They can cause cardiac dysfunction in patients with cardiac conduction problems or when used in combination with other medications that have cardiac effects and predisposes to ventricular tachyarrhythmia.

5. Empiric therapy refers to the selection of an antibiotic based on the most commonly encountered organisms at the site of the infection prior to obtaining culture results. If a patient is suspected of having a gram positive skin infection, empiric therapy might be based on the likelihood that the organism is *Staphylococcus*, and an antistaphylococcal penicillin might be prescribed while culture results are being obtained.

CHAPTER 27

Viral Infections

Matching I

Brand Names	Generic Names	Indication(s)	Route
1. Baraclude	d	HBV	PO
2. Copegus	l	HCV	PO
3. Cytovene	f	CMV	IV
4. Famvir	e	HSV	PO
5. Flumadine	m	Influenza A	PO
6. Hepsera	b	HBV	PO
7. Infergen	h	HCV	SQ
8. Intron A	g	HBV, HCV	IM, SQ
9. Pegasys	j	HBV, HCV	SQ
10. PegIntron	k	HBV	SQ
11. Rebetol	l	HCV	PO
12. Relenza	p	Influenza A, B	Inh
13. Sylatron	k	HBV	SQ
14. Tamiflu	i	Influenza A, B	PO
15. Valcyte	o	HSV	PO
16. Valtrex	n	HSV	PO
17. Virazole	l	RSV	Inh
18. Vistide	c	CMV	IV
19. Zirgan	f	CMV	oph
20. Zovirax	a	HSV	PO, IV, Top

Matching II

Brand Names	Generic Names	Mechanism of Action
1. Aptivus	s	PI
2. Crixivan	k	PI
3. Edurant	o	NNRTI
4. Emtriva	g	NRTI
5. Epivir	l	NRTI
6. Fuzeon	h	entry inhibitor

7. Intelence	i	NNRTI
8. Invirase	q	PI
9. Lexiva	j	PI
10. Norvir	p	PI
11. Prezista	c	PI
12. Rescriptor	d	NNRTI
13. Retrovir	t	NRTI
14. Reyataz	b	PI
15. Sustiva	f	NNRTI
16. Videx	e	NRTI
17. Viracept	m	PI
18. Viramune	n	NNRTI
19. Zerit	r	NRTI
20. Ziagen	a	NRTI

True or False

1. **T**

2. **F** Enteroviruses affect mainly the gastrointestinal tract.

3. **F** Herpesvirus infections cannot be cured by treatment with appropriate antiviral medications, but drugs with activity against them may reduce the severity of symptoms and frequency of their recurrence.

4. **T**

5. **F** Many viral infections can and should be treated with antiviral medications, but others, such as the common cold, viral gastroenteritis, and measles, are usually treated with supportive care instead.

6. **F** Neuraminidase inhibitors such as oseltamivir (Tamiflu) are effective against influenza if treatment is begun within 48 hours of the onset of symptoms.

7. **T**

8. **T**

9. **F** Additional antivirals are usually added to therapy with protease inhibitors for HIV because the development of resistant strains to PIs is so common.

10. **T**

Short Answer

1. Any three of the following:

   Some antivirals, such as maraviroc or enfuvirtide, block the attachment to and entry into the human cell. Others, like interferon alfa, block penetration of the viral particles into cellular contents. Amantadine and rimantadine block the uncoating of the influenza virus particle. NRTIs, NNRTIs, acyclovir, foscarnet, and entecavir interfere with viral nucleic acid synthesis. Protease inhibitors (see drugs in **Medication Table 27-2**) block synthesis of viral proteins, and neuraminidase inhibitors (zanamivir, oseltamivir) block the packaging and assembly of viral particles that spread to other body cells.

2. Medication guides for antivirals used in the treatment of hepatitis advise patients to avoid alcoholic beverages either because of drug interactions or because consuming alcohol can increase the liver damage caused by hepatitis.

3. Adamantines and neuraminidase inhibitors are indicated only for influenza. Most are given orally, but zanamivir (Relenza) is administered by inhalation.

4. Any three of the following:

   Cidofovir: intravenous; ganciclovir CAN be placed in the eye but may be administered IV; valganciclovir: oral; foscarnet: IV.

5. Antiretroviral therapy for HIV infection is complicated by the fact that regimens are complex and must be followed strictly, along with the near certainty that patients will experience side effects from treatment. There is currently no single drug treatment for HIV; all recommended regimens have at least three drugs from at least two different categories, such as two NNRTIs with a NRTI or two PIs with two NRTIs. If the dosage schedule is not followed strictly, viral resistance can develop, but the side effects can make this difficult.

CHAPTER 28

Fungal Infections

Matching

Brand Names	Generic Names	Route(s)	Dosage Form(s)
1. Abelcet	a	IV	Suspension
2. Ambisome	a	IV	Suspension
3. Amphotec	a	IV	Suspension
4. Cancidas	c	IV	Powder for recon
5. Diflucan	d	IV, PO	Tablet, solution
6. Eraxis	b	IV	Powder for recon
7. Monistat	g	V	Cream, suppository
8. Mycamine	f	IV	Powder for recon
9. Noxafil	h	PO	Suspension
10. Sporanox	e	PO	Capsule, solution
11. Terbinex	i	PO	Tablet
12. Vfend	j	IV, PO	Tablet, powder for recon

True or False

1. **F** A fungal cell resembles a human cell because it has a membrane-bound nucleus and organelles (unlike bacterial cells).

2. **F** Fungal cells, like bacterial cells, have a cell wall, but differences in its composition mean they are not susceptible to the same antibiotic medications used to treat bacterial infections.

3. **T**

4. **T**

5. **F** Azole antifungals, such as itraconazole, have many drug interactions because they interfere with liver metabolism of several medications.

6. **F** Voriconazole may be used in the treatment of *Aspergillus* fungal infections, but fluconazole has no activity against *Aspergillus*.

7. **T**

8. **F** For fungal infections of the skin, terbinafine is applied topically, but it is given orally for toenail infections because it accumulates in the nails.

9. **T**

10. **T**

Short Answer

1. Opportunistic pathogens are organisms that are not typically infectious but which are able to cause infection in an immunocompromised host. Although opportunistic pathogens seldom infect normal, healthy individuals, they can cause serious illness in patients who are in some state of immune compromise. Fungal infections are a commonly encountered type of opportunistic pathogen among immunocompromised patients. Fungi such as *Candida* and *Aspergillus* species tend to infect patients who are immunocompromised.

2. There are three lipid-based amphotericin B products; all are suspensions of liquid droplets and intended for IV administration. They have slightly different generic names (Abelcet is amphotericin B lipid, Ambisome is amphotericin B liposomal, and Amphotec is amphotericin B cholesteryl sulfate complex) and different dosing recommendations so they cannot be generically interchanged. Abelcet and Ambisome require an inline filter, and Amphotec must NOT be filtered.

3. Nystatin is not well absorbed into the body following oral administration so most of the dose included in the oral suspension remains in the mouth, throat, and gastrointestinal tract. Thus, the most common side effects from this preparation are stomach upset or diarrhea. Nystatin is also available as a topical cream, topical ointment, and a topical powder for the treatment of *Candida* skin infections.

4. Fluconazole is available as an oral tablet, oral solution, and a solution for intravenous administration. It is commonly utilized as oral therapy for a variety of uncomplicated *Candida* infections; because of its high oral bioavailability and long half-life, it can be administered for vaginal candidiasis as a one-time oral dose of 150 mg. The intravenous formulation is also commonly utilized for the treatment of more severe *Candida* infections such as bloodstream infections or infections of the central nervous system. In addition to its activity against a variety of *Candida* species, fluconazole is also active against a number of the endemic fungi and is sometimes used as an alternative agent in the treatment of these infections. However, fluconazole possesses no antifungal activity against *Aspergillus* species, and some species of *Candida* have developed resistance to fluconazole.

5. The term endemic fungal infections refers to those infections that are common only among certain populations or in certain regions. The three most important endemic fungal infections in the United States are *Histoplasma capsulatum* (generally found in the eastern United States, especially in the Ohio River Valley), *Coccidioides immitis* (occurring in the southwestern United States and northern Mexico), and *Blastomyces dermatitidis* (found in the eastern United States and Canada). These infections are transmitted through the inhalation of fungal spores. They typically cause pulmonary infections including pneumonia and pulmonary cavitations; however, the infections can disseminate to other parts of the body, chiefly in immunocompromised patients. Treatment of these infections generally involves treatment with antifungal agents but may also include surgical intervention.

CHAPTER 29

Immunobiologics

Matching I

Brand Names	Type of Infection(s)	Routes Other Than IM
1. Adacel	a, k, p	
2. BCG	q	percutaneous
3. Boostrix	a, k, p	
4. Engerix-B	d	
5. Fluarix	g	IM, intradermal
6. FluMist	g	intranasal
7. Fluzone	g	IM, intradermal
8. Gardasil	f	
9. Havrix	c	
10. Hiberix	b	
11. Menactra	i	
12. Menveo	i	
13. M-M-R II	h, j, n	
14. Pediarix	a, d, k, l, p	
15. Prevnar 13	o	
16. Recombivax HB	d	
17. Rotarix	m	oral
18. Vaqta	c	
19. Varivax	r	subQ
20. Zostavax	e	subQ

Matching II

Brand Names	Generic Names	Route(s)
1. Afinitor	f	PO
2. Atgam	a	IV
3. CellCept	g	IV, PO
4. Gengraf	e	PO
5. Hecoria	i	PO
6. Imuran	c	PO
7. Myfortic	g	IV, PO
8. Neoral	e	PO
9. Nulojix	d	IV
10. Prograf	i	IV, PO
11. Rapamune	h	PO
12. Sandimmune	e	IV, PO
13. Thymoglobulin	b	IV
14. Zortress	f	PO

True or False

1. **T**

2. **F** The immunity acquired after receiving an immune globulin is immediate but lasts only a few weeks or months.

3. **T**

4. **F** Although most vaccines are administered by injection, some (including typhoid, rotavirus, and cholera) can be given orally, and others (notably influenza) can be inhaled.

5. **F** Tetanus vaccinations should be repeated every 10 years, but influenza vaccinations should be received annually.

6. **T**

7. **F** Organ transplant patients receive immunosuppressive medications to prevent their immune systems from attacking the transplanted organ and causing rejection.

8. **F** Mycophenolate tablets and capsules must always be swallowed whole and should never be chewed or dissolved.

9. **T**

10. **T**

Short Answer

1. An immune globulin is an antibody or a preparation containing antibodies derived from a human or animal source that has been exposed to one or more antigens. Administration of immune globulins can confer passive immunity.

2. Most vaccines must be refrigerated or frozen continuously, and allowing them to reach a temperature that is outside the range in their labeling (thawing a frozen product, freezing one that should be kept at refrigerator temperatures, letting a product that must be kept cold to reach room temperature) can damage them irretrievably and cause failures of immunization that are not immediately apparent but can ultimately be deadly. Observing and maintaining the storage conditions on the labeling of each package is required at all times. Most vaccines must be shipped in an insulated container, and many have an enclosed temperature monitor to verify that they have not been exposed to temperatures outside their recommended storage ranges. When receiving vaccine products, technicians should examine the shipping container and contents for damage

and check the temperature monitor (if present). They should immediately place the products in the refrigerator or freezer at recommended temperatures.

3. Immunization can be accomplished by exposing (usually by injection, oral ingestion, or inhalation) people to killed or weakened versions of the pathogens that cause disease. Sometimes, the exposure is only to part of the pathogen (usually a bacterium or virus) — a part that is recognized as an antigen by the body but which cannot reproduce or cause infection. As a result of such exposures, the immune system develops memory cells that will recognize the parts of an active disease agent (like the ones to which it has been exposed), and the antibodies formed will circulate and be ready to attack an infective agent and prevent infection and illness before they can occur. The preparation containing killed or weakened pathogens is called a vaccine.

4. Postexposure prophylaxis refers to measures taken to prevent illness or infection after acute exposure of a nonimmune individual to a pathogen that can cause serious or fatal disease. This may include administration of specific immune sera/immunoglobulins. Examples include hepatitis B immune globulin administered to infants born of HBV-infected mothers or to healthcare workers with needlestick exposures and rabies immune globulin administered to a patient who has been bitten by a potentially rabid animal. Normal vaccines to produce active immunity against these antigens are available, but in cases such as these, immediate protection is needed to avoid infection or serious/fatal illness.

5. Cyclosporine is metabolized by the liver and has many drug interactions that can either increase blood levels (and risk of toxicity) or decrease them (chancing organ rejection). Some drugs can also have increased effects when taken with cyclosporine because cyclosporine inhibits the liver's metabolism of those medications.

CHAPTER 30

Cancer

Matching I

Brand Names	Generic Names	Type of Cancers
1. Abraxane	q	breast
2. Adriamycin	g	leukemia, lymphoma, breast, many others
3. Alimta	r	mesothelioma, lung
4. Arimidex	a	breast, colorectal
5. Camptosar	m	colorectal, lymphoma
6. Casodex	b	prostate
7. Doxil	h	multiple myeloma, ovarian
8. Eligard	o	prostate
9. Eloxatin	p	colorectal
10. Femara	n	breast
11. Gemzar	i	breast, lung, pancreatic, ovarian
12. Hydrea	k	leukemia, head and neck tumors
13. Ifex	l	testicular
14. Leukeran	e	leukemia
15. Lupron	o	prostate
16. Myleran	c	leukemia
17. Navelbine	s	lung
18. Taxotere	f	breast, prostate, lung
19. Xeloda	d	breast
20. Zoladex	j	prostate, breast

Matching II

Brand Names	Generic Names	Routes	Type of Cancer
1. Avastin	b	IV	colorectal, lung, glioblastoma, renal
2. Erbitux	c	IV	colorectal, squamous cell
3. Gleevec	f	PO	leukemia, GI
4. Herceptin	j	IV	breast, GI
5. Iressa	e	PO	lung
6. Proleukin	a	IV	renal cell, melanoma
7. Rituxan	h	IV	lymphoma, leukemia
8. Sutent	i	PO	GI, renal, pancreatic
9. Tarceva	d	PO	lung, pancreas
10. Yervoy	g	IV	melanoma

True or False

1. **T**

2. **F** Emetogenic potential refers to the tendency of a medication to cause nausea and vomiting.

3. **T**

4, **F** Vitamin supplements containing folic acid are often prescribed for patients taking permetrexed to reduce its toxicity.

5. **T**

6. **T**

7. **F** Vinca alkaloids are never administered intrathecally.

8. **F** Hormonal therapies like aromatase inhibitors are used not only in the treatment of life-threatening tumors, but for other conditions (including aromatase inhibitors for ovulation disorders or megestrol to stimulate appetite).

9. **F** Chemotherapies in liposomal or protein-bound forms are not generically equivalent to other dosage forms and may never be substituted without consultation.

10. **T**

Short Answer

1. Body surface area (BSA) is a measurement of the external area of the body, generally expressed in square meters (abbreviated m^2). It can be measured but is most often calculated from a patient's height and weight. Because it is thought to be a more accurate indicator of a patient's actual size than weight alone, it is often used in dose calculations for especially dangerous drugs that would require extra precision (like cancer chemotherapy).

2. Biological response modifiers (BRMs) are substances normally produced by the human body to direct processes and activities in the immune system. These agents alter the interaction between the body's immune system and cancer cells to boost, direct, or restore the body's ability to fight the disease. Interferons (IFNs) suppress cell proliferation and increase immune system activity against target cells. They are used in the treatment of some cancers, including hairy cell leukemia, melanoma, chronic myeloid leukemia, and AIDS-related Kaposi's sarcoma. Interleukins stimulate interferon production as well as increasing the activity of "killer" cells in the immune system. These actions can be directed against tumor cells.

3. A cytoprotective agent protects cells against damage from cytotoxins, including those administered as antineoplastic chemotherapy. Examples include mesna, which can protect the bladder from toxicities of ifosfamide, and dexrazoxane, which is a cytoprotective agent that reduces the damage by free radicals created in anthracycline exposure.

4. The antineoplastic agents discussed in this chapter are seldom used alone. A cancer chemotherapy regimen is a combination of medications in specific dose ranges and intervals designed to increase the likelihood of successful therapy, while decreasing the severity of the side effects. Medications from different groups, with different mechanisms of action, are chosen to attack the cancer cells in multiple ways, either simultaneously or sequentially.

5. Myelosuppression is an interference with the bone marrow's functions, especially production of blood cells and platelets and is one of the most common toxicities limiting the dose or continuation of therapy for antineoplastic agents. Neutrophils have a relatively short lifespan and are among the first type of cell to be depleted during therapy with myelosuppressive agents; when their count falls too low, patients suffer from neutropenia and are more susceptible to infection.

CHAPTER 31

Overview of the Skin and Topical Dosage Forms

Matching

Brand Names	Generic Ingredients	Indication
1. Alora	c	hormone replacement
2. Androderm	o	hormone replacement
3. Catapres-TTS	a	hypertension
4. Climara	c	hormone replacement
5. CombiPatch	d	hormone replacement
6. Daytrana	h	ADHD
7. Duragesic	f	pain
8. Emsam	n	depression
9. Estraderm	c	hormone replacement
10. Exelon	l	dementia
11. Flector	b	pain
12. Habitrol	i	smoking cessation
13. Lidoderm	g	pain
14. Minitran	i	angina
15. Nicoderm	i	smoking cessation
16. Nitro-Dur	j	angina
17. Ortho Evra	e	contraception
18. Oxytrol	k	overactive bladder
19. Transderm Scōp	m	motion sickness
20. Vivelle-Dot	c	hormone replacement

True or False

1. **T**

2. **F**   Topical dusting powders can cause irritation to the lungs if inhaled.

3. **F**   The transdermal route of administration is intended to provide a systemic effect for medications.

4. **T**

5. **F**   OTC topical products applied to the skin can cause drug overdoses, especially if used in excess or not according to the package directions.

6. **T**

7. **F**   Placement of transdermal patches should be rotated to minimize skin irritation.

8. **F**   Absorption of medications from transdermal patches is usually more steady and predictable compared with dosage forms given orally.

9. **T**

10. **T**

Short Answer

1. A local drug action is an effect directly at the site of application. An example would be application of a product to the skin for an effect ON the skin (like a sunscreen or anti-itch cream). A systemic action is one that comes from a drug in the bloodstream that has effects all over the body. An example might be a drug taken orally or administered intravenously but also includes medications administered for transdermal absorption (like the ones in this chapter's drug table).

2. Infants and children have a higher ratio of total body surface area (mostly skin) to body mass, placing them at risk for increased absorption of agents applied to the skin that may be systemically absorbed. Newborns may be harmed by application of common OTC preparations including rubbing alcohol, antiseptics, and pain relief products, and pharmacy technicians can remind parents who purchase such products to read the package labeling before using them.

3. Dosage forms for topical administration include:
   - Ointments: thick, oily, semisolid formulations that protect the skin surface and seal against water loss. A very thick ointment may be called a paste.
   - Creams: semisolids that are easier to apply and less thick than ointments; they wash with water.
   - Solutions: liquid preparations that contain a drug dissolved in a vehicle; less stable than semisolid dosage forms. Sometimes called lotions.
   - Gels: quick-drying, transparent semisolids that are water-soluble and provide quick drug release.
   - Powders: finely divided, dry solid dosage forms that can be sprinkled or dusted.

4. Pharmacy technicians can remind patients using transdermal patches to closely follow the supplied directions for patch placement, removal, storage, and disposal. These include being sure the skin on which they are placed is clean and dry, removing the old patch before placing a new one, never using a patch that has been cut or torn, and determining whether used patches should be flushed down the toilet or discarded in the trash.

5. Cutting or tearing a transdermal patch may lead to a change in the way the drug is released, increasing drug absorption and adverse or toxic effects.

CHAPTER 32
Treatment of Dermatologic Disorders

Matching I

Brand Names	Generic Names	Oral Administration
1. Aczone	e	
2. Akne-Mycin	g	
3. Amnesteem	h	PO
4. Avage	i	
5. Avita	j	
6. Benzac AC	b	
7. BenzaShave	b	
8. Benziq	b	
9. Brevoxyl	b	
10. Claravis	h	PO
11. ClindaMax	d	
12. Desquam-X	b	
13. Differin	a	
14. Epiduo	c	
15. Ery-Tab	g	PO
16. Evoclin	d	
17. Pacnex	b	
18. PanOxyl	b	
19. Renova	j	
20. Retin-A	j	
21. Sotret	h	PO
22. Tazorac	i	
23. Tretin-X	j	
24. Triaz	b	
25. Vibramycin	f	PO

Matching II

Brand Names	Generic Names	Dosage Form
1. Aclovate	a	0.05% cream, ointment
2. ApexiCon	g	ointment, cream
3. Clobex	c	shampoo, spray, solution, ointment
4. Cloderm	d	cream, lotion
5. Cordran	j	cream, lotion, tape
6. Cormax	c	solution, ointment, cream, gel
7. Cutivate	k	cream, ointment
8. DesOwen	e	cream, ointment, lotion, foam
9. Elocon	p	cream, ointment, lotion
10. Halog	l	cream, ointment, solution
11. Kenalog	q	cream, ointment, lotion
12. Locoid	n	ointment, cream
13. Luxiq	b	foam
14. Olux	c	foam
15. Synalar	h	0.025% cream, ointment
16. Temovate	c	solution, ointment, cream, gel
17. Topicort	f	0.25% cream, ointment gel
18. Ultravate	m	0.05% cream, ointment
19. Vanos	i	0.1% cream
20. Westcort	o	ointment

Matching III

Brand Names	Generic Names	Indications
1. Altabax	q	bacterial infection
2. AmLactin	b	dermatitis
3. Aveeno	j	dermatitis
4. Bactroban	m	bacterial infection
5. Balmex	v	dermatitis
6. Burow's	a	dermatitis
7. Calcitrene	e	psoriasis
8. Desitin	v	dermatitis
9. Dovonex	e	psoriasis
10. Dritho-creme	c	psoriasis
11. Ertaczo	r	fungal infection
12. Exelderm	s	fungal infection
13. Ionil-T	i	psoriasis
14. Lac-Hydrin	b	dermatitis
15. Loprox	h	fungal infection
16. Lotrimin Ultra	d	fungal infection
17. Mentax	d	fungal infection
18. Micatin	l	fungal infection
19. Neosporin	n	bacterial infection
20. Nizoral	k	fungal infection
21. Oxistat	o	fungal infection
22. Penlac	h	fungal infection
23. Polysporin	p	bacterial infection
24. Taclonex	f	psoriasis
25. Tinactin	t	fungal infection
26. Tucks	u	dermatitis
27. Vectical	g	psoriasis
28. Xolegel	k	fungal infection
29. Zeasorb-AF	l	fungal infection
30. Zithranol	c	psoriasis

True or False

1. **F** Several OTC acne treatments based on benzoyl peroxide may be effective and are recommended by pharmacists and physicians.

2. **T**

3. **F** Diaper rash is a form of irritant contact dermatitis.
4. **T**
5. **F** Areas of the skin exposed to poison oak should be washed with regular soap and water to remove the allergen. Harsh cleaners should not be used.
6. **F** Oral antibiotics may be necessary to treat some skin infections, especially cellulitis.
7. **T**
8. **F** Treatment for athlete's foot should be continued for 2 to 4 weeks, even if symptoms disappear earlier.
9. **T**
10. **T**

Short Answer

1. The biggest danger of oral isotretinoin therapy is the high risk of serious birth defects (including craniofacial, cardiovascular, thymus, parathyroid, and CNS structure malformations) to children born of women who took it during any phase of pregnancy. It may also cause spontaneous abortion and premature delivery. The iPledge Program was developed to prevent this from occurring, and the pharmacy is required to verify that the patient has had a (negative) pregnancy test within 7 days before picking up a prescription.

2. Biologic response modifiers are much more expensive than other psoriasis therapies, which is one reason they are not prescribed for cases in which other agents would be as effective. A more important reason is that the biologic response modifiers impair the immune system and place patients at a higher risk for serious infection and possibly cancer.

3. The two types of contact dermatitis are irritant and allergic. Irritant contact dermatitis is a result of skin exposure to substances that cause damage to the dermal layer. Initial treatment is by cleansing the affected area. Symptomatic treatment is with astringents (aluminum acetate, calamine) and topical corticosteroids. Allergic contact dermatitis can occur after direct skin contact with an allergen (fomite) or after inhalation of the allergen, leading to an allergic reaction and an inflammatory response in the dermal layer. Initial treatment is similar to that for the irritant type, but more serious cases may be treated with systemic (prescription) corticosteroids, usually oral but, if necessary, by the intravenous or intramuscular routes.

4. The first-line treatment for cold sores is the use of skin protectant, such as lip balm, to keep the cold sore moist and prevent cracking. The only topical antiviral recommended for cold sores is docosanol, but it is only useful if application begins at the first sign of a cold sore, before it erupts.

5. Many skin conditions can be managed with OTC products, but others require a physician's care. Among those that can be self-treated, it is often difficult, but important, to identify which condition to treat so that the right products are chosen. The pharmacist can counsel patients in choosing properly (or refer them to their physicians), and technicians can be sure that patients purchasing OTC preparations have had appropriate consultation before attempting self-treatment.

CHAPTER 33

Ophthalmic Medications

Matching I

Brand Names	Generic Names	Class
1. Alphagan	d	sympathomimetic
2. Azopt	e	carbonic anhydrase inhibitor
3. Betagan	h	beta blocker
4. Betoptic-S	b	beta blocker
5. Iopidine	a	sympathomimetic
6. Isopto carpine	j	cholinergic
7. Lumigan	c	prostaglandin
8. Miostat	f	cholinergic
9. Optipranolol	i	beta blocker
10. Timoptic	k	beta blocker
11. Travatan Z	l	prostaglandin
12. Trusopt	g	carbonic anhydrase inhibitor

Matching II

Brand Names	Generic Names	Class	OTC
1. Alaway	j	antihistamine	OTC
2. Alocril	o	mast cell stabilizer	
3. Alomide	l	mast cell stabilizer	
4. AzaSite	b	antibiotic	
5. Bepreve	c	mast cell stabilizer	
6. Besivance	d	antibiotic	
7. Bleph-10	r	antibiotic	
8. Ciloxan	e	antibiotic	
9. Claritin eye	j	antihistamine	OTC
10. Elestat	g	antihistamine	
11. Emadine	f	antihistamine	

12. Gentak	i	antibiotic	
13. Iquix	k	antibiotic	
14. Moxeza	m	antibiotic	
15. Natacyn	n	antifungal	
16. Ocuflox	p	antibiotic	
17. Optivar	a	antihistamine	
18. Pataday	q	antihistamine	
19. Patanol	q	antihistamine	
20. Tobrex	s	antibiotic	
21. Vigamox	m	antibiotic	
22. Viroptic	t	antiviral	
23. Zaditor	j	antihistamine	OTC
24. Zymaxid	h	antibiotic	
25. Zyrtec itchy eye	j	antihistamine	OTC

Matching III

Brand Names	Generic Names	Corticosteroid/ NSAID
1. Acular	d	NSAID
2. Acuvail	d	NSAID
3. Alrex	e	corticosteroid
4. Durezol	b	corticosteroid
5. Flarex	c	corticosteroid
6. FML	c	corticosteroid
7. Lotemax	e	corticosteroid
8. Maxidex	a	corticosteroid
9. Nevanac	f	NSAID
10. Omnipred	g	corticosteroid
11. Pred Forte	g	corticosteroid
12. Vexol	h	corticosteroid

True or False

1. **F** Eye drops for glaucoma all work by decreasing intraocular pressure, but they do so in different ways, so it is common for a patient to have a prescription for more than one at a time.

2. **T**

3. **F** Treatments for macular degeneration are not administered as eye drops, but are usually given as an injection either into the eye itself or intravenously, depending on the agent.

4. **T**

5. **F** Ophthalmic antihistamines seldom cause drowsiness the way oral antihistamines do.

6. **T**

7. **T**

8. **F** Contact lenses should be removed before administration of medicated eye drops and left out for at least 15 minutes afterward (or longer).

9. **T**

10. **F** Dry eyes can often be treated with prescription OTC lubricants.

Short Answer

1. Eye tissue is much more sensitive than ear tissue, so eye drops must be specifically buffered and formulated to avoid burning, stinging, redness, and/or swelling. These formulations are usually effective in the ear as well, but otic drops administered in the eye may cause the problems mentioned in the first sentence.

2. Ophthalmic suspensions should be rolled between the hands before administration to resuspend particles of active ingredients that may have settled. Resuspension by shaking should be avoided because it could cause formation of bubbles, which would interfere with proper administration.

3. Mydriasis is dilation (enlargement) of the pupil. This is helpful during eye examinations in which the back of the eye is to be examined because the opening stays bigger. Mydriatic agents used in eye exams include atropine, homatropine, and cyclopentolate, all of which may cause temporary vision changes like blurry vision or difficulty in focusing.

4. Classes of glaucoma treatment agents include the following (question asks for two of these):

   - Beta blockers; carbonic anhydrase inhibitors; alpha sympathomimetics: reduce IOP by reducing production (amount) of aqueous humor.
   - Prostaglandin analogues; brimonidine (alpha sympathomimetic): reduce IOP by increasing outflow of aqueous humor.
   - Cholinergics: reduce IOP by causing miosis (decreased pupil size), increasing outflow of aqueous humor.

5. The most common side effects of anti-infective eye drops are burning and stinging in the eye after administration.

CHAPTER 34

Ear Medications

Matching

Brand Names	Ingredients	Status	Indication
1. Auro-DRI	e	OTC	water-clogging
2. Auroguard	a	OTC	anesthetic
3. Cipro HC	c	RX	otitis
4. Coly-Mycin S	d	RX	otitis
5. Debrox	b	OTC	excess cerumen
6. Murine	b	OTC	excess cerumen
7. Otix	b	OTC	excess cerumen
8. Swim-EAR	e	OTC	water-clogging

True or False

1. **F** Carbamide peroxide ear drops are not indicated to treat children under the age of 12 for excess earwax unless they have been prescribed by a physician.

2. **T**

3. **F** Children with otitis media are usually treated with orally administered antibiotics.

4. **F** Excessive or impacted cerumen is the most common cause of hearing loss.

5. **T**

Short Answer

1. Ear candles are hollow candles made of a fabric tube soaked in beeswax or paraffin or a combination of both. One end is burned while the other is inserted into the ear canal. The pharmacist is unlikely to recommend their use because the FDA has warned patients that they can cause serious injuries including burns, broken eardrums, and blockage of the ear canal.

2. Cancer chemotherapy drugs, especially those containing platinum, can cause tinnitus and hearing loss that can present immediately or up to several months after finishing treatment. Typically, the hearing loss with platinum chemotherapeutic drugs affects both ears and is permanent. Loop diuretics (such as furosemide) are more likely to cause permanent hearing loss in patients with decreased kidney function and those receiving aminoglycosides. Aspirin in high doses (more than 12 325-mg tablets daily) can cause tinnitus and temporary hearing loss. Quinine can also cause temporary hearing loss.

3. To properly administer eardrops, the head should be tilted toward the opposite shoulder. The auricle should be pulled so that the canal is open and visible. Drops should be administered into the canal with the dropper as far into the canal as possible without touching the canal. Patients should lie on their sides for 20 minutes or place a cotton ball blocking the ear canal to maximize drug exposure.

CHAPTER 35

Mouth, Throat, and Nose Medications

Matching I

Brand Names	Ingredients	Indications	Actions
1. Anbesol	a	P	local anesthetic
2. Cepastat	e	P	local anesthetic
3. Chloraseptic	e	P	local anesthetic
4. Gly-Oxide	b	I	anti-inflammatory
5. Orajel	a	P	local anesthetic
6. Peridex	c	G	antibacterial
7. Periogard	c	G	antibacterial
8. Peroxyl	d	I	antibacterial
9. Xylocaine	f	P	local anesthetic

Matching II

Brand Names	Ingredients	Route	Class/Action
1. Afrin	l	X	decongestant
2. Allegra	h	Y	antihistamine
3. Astelin	a	X	antihistamine
4. Astepro	a	X	antihistamine
5. Benadryl	g	Y	antihistamine
6. Benzedrex	n	X	decongestant
7. Chlor-Trimeton	c	Y	antihistamine
8. Clarinex	f	Y	antihistamine
9. Claritin	j	Y	antihistamine
10. NasalCrom	e	X	mast cell stabilizer
11. Neo-Synephrine	m	X	decongestant

12. Privine	k	X	decongestant
13. Sudafed	o	Y	decongestant
14. Sudafed PE	m	Y	decongestant
15. Tavist	d	Y	antihistamine
16. Tyzine	p	X	decongestant
17. Xyzal	i	Y	antihistamine
18. Zyrtec	b	Y	antihistamine

True or False

1. **T**

2. **F** Thrush is a fungal infection that must be treated with a prescription antifungal medication.

3. **F** Local anesthetics for mouth and throat pain may cause methemoglobinemia, a dangerous condition, if overused.

4. **T**

5. **F** Rebound congestion refers to a return of congestion occurring after overuse (usually 3 days or more) of decongestant nasal drops.

6. **T**

7. **F** Colds are viral infections that can be managed but not cured using antihistamines and nasal decongestants.

8. **T**

9. **T**

10. **F** OTC products for cough and cold symptoms must be used cautiously with medications for pain relief, including those obtained with a prescription, because many contain duplicate ingredients, especially acetaminophen, so patients may receive an overdose.

Short Answer

1. An expectorant works by causing an increase in respiratory tract secretions, thus increasing the volume and thinning the mucus there. This makes it easier to cough mucus up. This will work best when patients consume increased amounts of water while taking an expectorant product.

2. A dry, hacking cough is often treated by suppressing it with an antitussive medication, such as dextromethorphan, an OTC remedy. A productive cough, however, serves a purpose by clearing the respiratory passages and should be treated by "encouraging" it with an expectorant. This helps thin the mucus, making it easier to clear, along with plenty of water. Antitussives may prevent this clearing, but they can be used at night if the cough is preventing the patient from sleeping.

3. Patients with high blood pressure and/or those taking antihypertensive medications should ask the pharmacist for help in choosing a decongestant because many of the orally administered products can cause increases in blood pressure. The pharmacist may recommend a nasally administered decongestant instead because these act locally and are less likely to affect the blood pressure (but should not be used for more than 3 consecutive days). Other patients for whom special cautions are recommended are children. Even though they are available without a prescription, many cold products contain ingredients such as decongestants and antihistamines and are not to be used in children under the age of 4. The pharmacist will probably recommend a pediatric-specific product or a visit to the pediatrician.

4. Oral decongestants and antihistamines are convenient to administer, and many are available OTC. They may cause systemic side effects (like blood pressure elevation with decongestants or drowsiness with antihistamines). Nasal administration is sometimes difficult or inconvenient but is less likely to cause systemic side effects. Nasal decongestants, however, can be administered only for a short period because they may cause rebound congestion. Nasal antihistamine drops are available only by prescription.

5. Federal law limits the amount of pseudoephedrine that can be purchased by an individual and requires that purchasers show identification. Many states have additional laws and rules regarding this ingredient. The reason these have been put into place is that pseudoephedrine can be used in the illegal manufacture of methamphetamine.